INTRODUCTION TO
EPIDEMIOLOGY

INTRODUCTION TO
EPIDEMIOLOGY

▼

Donald B. Stone
University of Illinois at Urbana-Champaign

Warwick R. Armstrong
University of Illinois at Urbana-Champaign

David M. Macrina
University of Alabama at Birmingham

Joseph W. Pankau
Oklahoma State University

▲

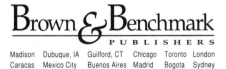

Brown & Benchmark
PUBLISHERS

Madison   Dubuque, IA   Guilford, CT   Chicago   Toronto London
Caracas   Mexico City   Buenos Aires Madrid   Bogota   Sydney

Book Team

Publisher *Bevan O'Callaghan*
Managing Editor *Ed Bartell*
Developmental Editor *Megan Rundel*
Publishing Services Coordinator *Peggy Selle*
Proofreading Coordinator *Carrie Barker*
Visual Editor *Rachel Imsland*
Production Manager *Beth Kundert*
Production/Costing Manager *Sherry Padden*
Visuals/Design Freelance Specialist *Mary L. Christianson*
Marketing Manager *Pamela S. Cooper*
Copywriter *M. J. Kelly*

Basal Text *10/12 Palatino*
Display Type *Helvetica*
Typesetting System *Macintosh™ QuarkXPress™*
Paper Stock *50# Solutions*
Production Services *Shepherd, Inc.*

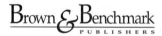

President and Chief Executive Officer *Thomas E. Doran*
Vice President of Production and Business Development *Vickie Putman*
Vice President of Sales and Marketing *Bob McLaughlin*
Director of Marketing *John Finn*

A Times Mirror Company

Cover design by Lesiak/Crampton Design, Inc.

Cover image © Ken Eward/BioGrafx/Science Source, Photo Researchers, Inc.

Cover image: Hantaviruses, agents of hemorrhagic fever, bud from the surface of a cultured kidney cell in this optical density plot made from a TEM. These viruses typically measure 100–200 nanometers in diameter. This image was produced from an electron micrograph provided by the CDC.

Copyedited by Shepherd, Inc.; proofread by Janet Reuter

Library of Congress Catalog Card Number: 95–76516

ISBN 0–697–12289–1

Printed in the United States of America by Times Mirror Higher Education Group, Inc., 2460 Kerper Boulevard, Dubuque, IA 52001

10 9 8 7 6 5 4 3 2 1

CONTENTS

PREFACE

This text is intended for introductory courses in epidemiology for undergraduate students enrolled in the health sciences or allied fields. The principles and concepts presented here should provide the necessary background for understanding the basics of epidemiological activity and classical epidemiological investigations. Epidemiology can be considered an applied science because it derives some of its concepts, methods, and knowledge from other disciplines, such as statistics, sociology, and microbiology. By applying knowledge from a range of disciplines, epidemiologists are able to more adequately study disease, wellness, and other health-related events in populations. Epidemiologists are also concerned with logical reasoning. They derive scientific inferences by observing disease occurrence and related health events in population groups.

We hope that our text will serve to stimulate students to enroll in additional courses in epidemiology and to consider the possibility of a future career in the field. There is a great need for trained epidemiologists in preventive medicine, to combat our present and newly emerging health problems. It is through an understanding of epidemiology that scientists, health planners, physicians, health educators, and allied health specialists can prepare to deal with the public health challenges of the future.

We would like to express our appreciation to the staff of the Centers for Disease Control and Prevention and the National Center for Health Statistics for providing materials and health data. For assistance with typing and clerical support, we are indebted to Kathy Lynn for her many hours of dedication, efficiency, and good humor.

As with any major undertaking, this text represents the combined efforts of many people. The authors wish to express their sincere appreciation to the many health professionals who provided constructive reviews and ideas to be included in the finished project. Also, we would like to thank Ed Bartell, Executive Managing Editor, Brown & Benchmark, for overseeing the project and for his persistence and patience; Kim

Olson, freelance developmental editor, and Laura Lenz, Shepherd, Inc., for their attention to detail during book development and talented skills in the production phase; and to the many other staff members who contributed their time and talent.

Finally, we owe our wives, Sue, Jocelyn, Nancy, and Mary, and our families a debt of gratitude for their unfailing support and encouragement. To all of you, a special thanks.

CHAPTER 1

The Scope of Epidemiology

Introduction

We are faced with an ever increasing number of questions about our health. Questions such as the following confront us on a daily basis: Is drinking decaffeinated coffee better for my health than regular coffee? Should I eat oat bran to lower my cholesterol? Will two glasses of wine a day provide protection from a heart attack? Are chemical pesticides on the fruit I eat harmful to my health? Can AIDS be transmitted to a baby from its infected mother by breast milk?

Over twenty-five years have elapsed since the Surgeon General's report, *Healthy people* (HHS 1979), attempted to articulate a government policy on improving the health status of our population. The report urged individuals to take a more responsible role in making healthy life-style choices. It is projected that in the 1990s, more than ever before, people will have to contend with the increasing explosion of information on all subjects, as predicted in the best-selling *Megatrends, 2000*. This book and many others point out that health will remain one of the most popular topics, as the enthusiasm for personal health improvement continues to expand within our society. Not only will questions of personal health life-style be important in the coming years, but questions of governmental health policy—such as those concerning pollution control and health-care delivery—will need to be addressed if we are to enhance the health of our citizenry. On an international scale as well, the recurring issues of hunger, sanitation, and communicable disease control will continue to face those concerned with health.

We might be tempted to think of ourselves as unique, because we have the opportunity to deal with all of these questions. In fact, however, we share with our ancestors the quest to understand what is happening around us and the degree to which our experiences affect our health. Humans have always had a need to identify, understand, and use a logical method both for answering the compelling health questions of the day and for initiating new ones.

Epidemiology is considered the fundamental science of public health. It is: (1) A quantitative basic science that focuses on a working knowledge of probability, statistics, and research methods; (2) a method of causal reasoning based on formulating and testing hypotheses pertaining to the occurrence and prevention of morbidity and mortality; and (3) a tool for concerted action to promote and protect the public's health, based on science, causal reasoning, and a dose of practical common sense (Cates 1982).

Definitions of Epidemiology

The definition of the word *epidemiology* comes from the Greek words *epi*, meaning "on or upon," *demos* meaning "people," and *logos* meaning "the study of."

Several definitions of the term epidemiology are useful to consider. Let us examine these definitions in order to identify the meaning of the term and to begin to develop a sense of the reasoning process that the practice of epidemiology entails. Some definitions of the term include the following:

1. "Epidemiology is the study of the distribution and determinants of health related states or events in specified populations, and the application of this study to the control of health problems" (Last 1992).
2. "Epidemiology is the study of the distribution of a disease or physiological condition in human populations and of the factors that influence this distribution" (Lilienfeld 1976).
3. "Epidemiology is the description and explanation of the differences in occurrence of events of medical concern in subgroups of a population, where the population has been subdivided according to some characteristic believed to influence the occurrence of the event" (Stallones 1971).
4. "Epidemiology is the study of the prevalence and dynamics of stages of health in populations" (Frerichs and Neutra 1978).

Each of these definitions suggests that the practice of epidemiology involves fundamental activities, whether we are health professionals or individuals making health decisions in our daily lives. At this point in our study of epidemiology, these activities might be described as observation, enumeration, and the determination of the nature of relationships between items. Put more simply, the practice of epidemiology involves taking note of what is going on around us, counting the items of which we are taking note, and attempting to draw some conclusions regarding the nature of any potential relationships we might discover. Subsequently, we might also be involved in determining the implications of the relationships we have identified.

Methods of Epidemiology

Epidemiology uses several methods or tools to study public health. The four basic methods are: public health surveillance, disease investigation, analytic studies, and program evaluation. All of these methods are necessary for contributing to the promotion of the public's health.

Public Health Surveillance

Surveillance involves the systematic collection, analysis, integration, and dissemination of health data on an ongoing basis (Thacker 1988). The major sources or kinds of data relevant to disease surveillance include the following:

1. Mortality reports
2. Morbidity reports
3. Epidemic reports
4. Reports of epidemic investigations
5. Reports of laboratory investigations
6. Reports of case investigations
7. Special surveys (e.g., hospital admissions, **serologic**, disease registers)
8. Information on animal reservoirs and vectors
9. Demographic data
10. Environmental data

Serologic–analysis of the properties and actions of blood serums.

Public health agencies use surveillance activities to monitor the health of their communities. The surveillance activities provide a factual basis from which agencies can establish priorities, plan programs, and take the necessary actions to promote and protect the health of their citizens (*Principles of Epidemiology 1992*).

Disease Investigation

The primary objective of a disease outbreak investigation is to control and prevent further disease. Typically, a disease outbreak investigation involves the accomplishment of the following objectives:

1. Establishing or verifying the diagnosis of reported cases and identifying the specific **etiological** agent responsible.
2. Confirming that an outbreak or an epidemic exists.
3. Describing the cases in the epidemic or outbreak according to the variables of time, place, and person.
4. Identifying the source of the agent and its mode of transmission, including the specific vehicles, vectors, and routes that may have been involved.
5. Identifying susceptible populations that are at an increased risk of exposure to the agent.

Etiological–dealing with the causes or origins of disease.

In some cases, further investigation may be necessary, depending on how much is known about the cause, source, and mode of transmission of the agent.

Analytic Studies

Epidemiologists need to be familiar with the design, conduct, analysis, and interpretive aspects of an analytic study. They need to consider the appropriate study design, writing, justifications and protocols, sample sizes, criteria for subject selection (e.g., choosing controls), questionnaires, and numerous other items that are part of the study plan.

The proper conduct of a study requires securing appropriate clearances and approvals, abstracting records, tracking down and interviewing subjects, collecting and handling specimens, and managing the data.

Study analysis begins with describing the characteristics of the subjects and progresses to calculating rates, creating comparative tables (e.g., risk ratios and odds ratios), doing tests of statistical significances (e.g., chi-square), establishing confidence intervals, and the like. Many epidemiological studies require more advanced analytic techniques, such as stratified analysis, regression, and modeling.

Interpretation involves putting the findings of a study into perspective and making appropriate recommendations to the proper authorities.

Evaluation

The evaluation of control and prevention measures is another responsibility of epidemiologists. Evaluation often addresses both effectiveness and efficiency. *Effectiveness* refers to the ability of a program to produce the intended or expected results in the field. Effectiveness differs from *efficacy*, which is the ability to produce results under *ideal* conditions. Finally, *efficiency* refers to the ability of a program to produce the intended results with a minimum expenditure of time and resources. The evaluation of an immunization program, for example, might compare the stated efficacy with the field effectiveness of the program, and it might assess the efficiency with which the acceptable results are achieved (*Principles of Epidemiology* 1992).

Uses of Epidemiology

For the student of health sciences, the rationale for a thorough understanding of the principles of epidemiology may seem readily apparent. There are many good reasons for having an organized and systematic method for studying the many aspects of public health. This is particularly true for health practitioners, such as health planners, administrators, and educators, who need an understanding of the nature of health problems, their causes, and potential solutions. As we will see in subsequent discussions within this text, the fundamental processes of epidemiological investigation have not always been the basis on which individual or societal health decisions were made.

Planning Policies and Programs

To determine appropriate health policies and to properly plan programs, public health officials must assess the health of the population or community they serve. They need to determine whether health services are available, accessible, effective, and efficient. In order to accomplish these tasks, certain questions need to be answered. For instance: What are the actual and potential health problems in the community? Where are they located? What are the characteristics of the population at risk? Are some health problems declining or increasing?

Epidemiological methods properly applied to these problems can provide answers, so that health personnel can make informed decisions and establish appropriate health policies.

Making Individual Decisions

As we indicated earlier, people may not realize that they use epidemiological information in their daily lives. For example, when people decide to have steamed rice instead of french fries or walk two miles to work instead of using their car, they may have been influenced by epidemiology studies reported in the media. Many studies continue to document the role of exercise and proper diet in reducing the risk of heart disease and other illnesses in a population.

Completing the Clinical Picture

Epidemiologists can contribute to the physicians' understanding of the clinical picture and the natural history of disease. For example, a unique hantavirus has been identified as the cause of an outbreak of respiratory illness, hantavirus pulmonary **syndrome** (HPS), first recognized in the southwestern central states in May 1993. Epidemiological studies have confirmed that this infection can be transmitted when infective saliva or excretion are inhaled as aerosols produced directly from rodent reservoirs. Transmission can also occur when dried materials contaminated by rodent excreta are disturbed, directly introduced into broken skin, introduced into the **conjunctivae**, or possibly ingested in contaminated food or water. Persons have also become infected after being bitten by rodents (CDC 1993). The Centers for Disease Control and Prevention (CDCP) is now assisting state health departments in other ongoing investigations of the hantavirus.

Epidemiology enables us to do many things in regard to public health.

1. To study the history of the health of the population and of the rise and fall of diseases and changes in their characteristics.

Syndrome–a group of signs and symptoms which, when considered together, characterize a disease or other type of illness.
Conjunctivae– mucous membrane lining the inner surface of the eyelids and covering the front part of the eyeball.

Prevalence–all cases of a disease in a population, both old and new.
Incidence–the number of new cases of a disease.
Morbidity–any departure, subjective or objective, from a state of physiological or psychological well being, i.e., illness.
Mortality–death, statistics on death.

2. To diagnose the health of the community and the conditions of people, and to measure the present dimensions and distribution of ill health in terms of **prevalence, incidence,** and **morbidity** and **mortality**.
3. To study the effects of health services with a view to their improvement; to describe needs and demands, and the current effectiveness of services, utilization, drugs, etc.
4. To estimate, from group experiences, individuals' risks and the changes of diseases, accidents, and defects.
5. To complete the clinical picture of a chronic and infectious disease and to describe its natural history.
6. To identify syndromes by describing the distribution, association, and dissociation of clinical phenomena in the population.
7. To search for causes of health and disease by studying the incidence in different groups, defined in terms of their composition, experience, behavior, and interaction with the environment.

Searching for Causes

A significant amount of epidemiological research is devoted to a search for causes, factors that influence one's risk of disease. Often the goal is to identify a cause, so that appropriate public health action might be taken. It has been said that epidemiology can never *prove* a causal relationship between an exposure and a disease. Nevertheless, epidemiology often provides enough information to support effective action. Examples include John Snow's removal of a water pump handle in a cholera epidemic and the withdrawal of a specific brand of tampon that was linked by epidemiologists to toxic shock syndrome before the exact nature of the causative agents were identified. Just as often, epidemiology and laboratory science converge to provide the evidence needed to establish causation. For example, a team of epidemiologists was able to identify a variety of risk factors during an outbreak of pneumonia among persons attending the American Legion Convention in Philadelphia in 1976. However, the outbreak was not "solved" until the Legionnaires' bacillus was identified in the laboratory almost six months later (*Principles of Epidemiology* 1992).

Preventing Disease

Epidemiology has been referred to as the "science of prevention" (Green 1990). The application of epidemiological data allows us to take and plan actions in terms of preventing or dealing with disease and other undesirable health conditions. One paradigm of prevention separates activities into three distinct levels, the primary, secondary, and tertiary levels of prevention.

The *primary* level of prevention is activity designed to prevent undesirable conditions and their precursors from occurring (such as in vaccination programs). Thus, in the primary prevention category we could place activities such as eating a healthy diet to prevent cardiovascular disease, educating children not to smoke as a means of preventing tobacco-related lung disease, and jogging as a means of promoting cardiovascular health. Thus, changing the behavior of individuals becomes an important mechanism for primary prevention.

Secondary prevention emphasizes the early recognition of disease and other undesirable conditions in order that initial intervention efforts might begin. The periodic screening of schoolchildren at selective grade levels for visual, dental, and hearing abnormalities is an example of a secondary prevention action. The screenings are designed to identify children who exhibit early signs and symptoms in order to provide assistance as early in the diseases as possible. Hypertension and cholesterol screening in shopping malls are two more examples of secondary prevention activities popular in today's society. While secondary prevention activities may require assistance from others, such as health professionals (e.g., the taking of blood for cholesterol screening), an increasing number of testing kits and procedures allow individuals to practice secondary prevention in their own homes. Some secondary prevention activities, such as breast self-examination and testicular self-examination for cancer, require knowledge, skill, and practice on the part of the individual. Other secondary prevention activities require additional materials, which can be purchased at most drug stores. The rise in popularity of home-testing kits, such as those to detect pregnancy, fecal occult blood, and sugar in the blood, are evidence of the increasing interest of the public in secondary prevention.

Tertiary prevention is activity that attempts to restore and rehabilitate the individual, so far as possible, to the **premorbid** state. Tertiary prevention programs, such as Alcoholics Anonymous and cardiac rehabilitation, are efforts to restore individuals with undesirable conditions and diseases to their health status prior to the onset of disease or injury.

Premorbid–before entering the morbid state or illness.

Each of these levels of prevention rely on the techniques of epidemiological investigation both to assess the need for intervention and to monitor the effectiveness of subsequent treatment.

Epidemiology and the Objectives for the Nation

The application of epidemiological methods assists us as individuals in making healthful decisions regarding our life-style choices. On the national level as well, the practice of epidemiology enables us to assess the current status of our nation's health and to set future goals for improvement.

The recent history of health promotion reveals several governmental policy and planning documents that implicitly use epidemiological techniques. Epidemiological methods have been used to assess current health conditions, to suggest intervention strategies, and to formulate goal statements toward which intervention strategies might be targeted.

Evidence of the epidemiological methods are inherent within the pages of many of the documents considered to be landmarks in the development of health promotion. For example, governmental policy statements in the 1970s on the health status of citizens in three nations (Canada, England, and the United States) encouraged individuals to examine the role that their health decisions played in determining their future health status. Each of the three documents—*A new perspective on the health of Canadians*, 1974, in Canada; *Prevention and health: Everybody's business*, 1976, in England; and *Healthy people*, 1979, in the United States—asked individuals and government planners to consider the epidemiological evidence linking life-style and health status. Each of the documents also called on individuals and governments to take action to improve individual and collective health.

Subsequently, within the United States, an additional planning document, *Promoting Health and Preventing Disease: Objectives for the Nation—1990*, established a definitive direction in the quest for improved health status. The *1990 Objectives*, as the document is often called, outlined specific goals for preventive services, health protection, and health promotion to be achieved by the year 1990. Each of the goals was justified by an accompanying rationale, which delineated the epidemiological data used in developing the goal statements. When we examine the areas included in the objectives (see Table 1.1) we gain a

TABLE 1.1 Components of the Areas of the 1990 Objectives for the Nation.

Health Content Area	Topical Subjects
1. Preventive services	High blood pressure control Family planning Pregnancy and infant health Immunization Sexually transmitted disease
2. Health protection	Toxic agent and radiation control Occupational health and safety Accident prevention and injury control Fluoridation and dental health Surveillance and control of infectious diease
3. Health promotion	Smoking and health Misuse of alcohol and drugs Nutrition Physical fitness and exercise Control of stress and violent behavior

Source: *Promoting health and preventing disease: Objectives for the nation—1990*, Washington: U.S. Department of Health and Human Services, 1980.

good idea of the breadth of health areas to which epidemiological investigation can be applied.

Summary

This chapter has delineated the broad scope of epidemiology and its applications for individual and societal health. The important methods of surveillance, disease investigation, analytic studies, and program evaluation were discussed as these pertain to the promotion of the public's health.

The concept of health decision making was introduced, and the numerous uses of epidemiology were discussed. In particular, the levels of prevention—primary, secondary, and tertiary—were outlined in relation to the need for intervention and monitoring.

Finally, several government publications were discussed, reflecting the current concern of governments with life-style changes and health promotion. Several of these reports were based on the application of epidemiological investigations.

Discussion Questions

1. Discuss why epidemiology is considered to be the fundamental science of public health.
2. Describe the four basic methods of epidemiology as they relate to promoting the health of the public.
3. What are the common uses of epidemiology in today's practice of public health?
4. Discuss the different levels of prevention that rely on epidemiological investigation.
5. How has epidemiology enabled us to assess the current status of our nation's health?

References

Cates, J. W. 1982. Epidemiology: Applying principle to clinical practice. *Contemporary Obstetrics/Gynecology* 20:147–161.

Centers for Disease Control, 1993. MMWR. Hantavirus infection—Southwestern United States—Interim recommendations for risk reduction. 42 (RR-11):2–13.

Freidman, G. 1974. *Primer of epidemiology.* New York: McGraw-Hill.

Frerichs, R., and R. Neutra. 1978. *Re: Definitions of epidemiology. American Journal of Public Health* 108:74.

Green, L. 1980. *Community health.* St. Louis: Times/Mirror Mosby.

Healthy people: The surgeon general's report on health promotion and disease prevention. Washington, U.S. Department of Health and Human Services, 1979.

Last, J. ed. 1992. *Dictionary of epidemiology,* 2nd ed. New York: Oxford University Press, 43.

Lilienfeld, D.E., and P. D. Stolley. 1994. *Foundations of epidemiology,* 3rd ed. New York: Oxford University Press.

Mausner, J., and S. Kramer. 1985. *Epidemiology: An introductory text*. Philadelphia: W. B. Saunders.

Principles of epidemiology. Atlanta, GA: U.S. Department of Health and Human Services, Centers for Disease Control, 1992.

Promoting health and preventing disease, objectives for the nation—1990, Washington: U.S. Department of Health and Human Services, 1980.

Promoting health/preventing disease, objectives for the year 2000. Washington: U.S. Department of Health and Human Services, 1989, (draft).

Stallones, R. 1980. To advance epidemiology. *Annual Review of Public Health* 1:69.

Thacker, S., and R. Berkelman. 1988. Public health surveillance in the United States. *Epidemiological Review* 10:164–190.

CHAPTER 2

The Historical Foundations of Epidemiology

Introduction

To gain some understanding of the origin and evolution of the science of epidemiology, it is necessary to briefly review some of the earlier concepts of health and disease that influenced human thought. Throughout history, humans have had to deal with the threats of disease, injury, and illness. These threats have long challenged human ingenuity, as we have attempted to devise methods to cope with these natural phenomena.

People's early ideas concerning health and illness involved the interaction of psychological, cultural, and social forces with their environment. Their basic beliefs concerning disease enabled them to accept or reject certain concepts pertaining to the origin and **pathogenesis** of disease and illness. Early civilizations analyzed illness in a subjective manner; their thoughts and actions were dominated by feelings, urges, desires, hopes, superstitions, and fears. Disease was perceived as being due to "spirit-like" forces or to factors that were **intrapsychic** in nature. People's perceptions of the world were sometimes distorted and perhaps overwhelmed by the more emotional aspects of their imaginations.

Under these circumstances, it is not surprising that many magical, supernatural, and unscientific methods were tried in order to treat illness and restore health. If the cure worked, no surprise was evidenced; if the method failed, something else could be tried. However, if the patient were restored to health, the remedy was usually credited with effecting the cure. Early attempts to treat sickness were generally rooted in supernatural beliefs and required only occasional successes to maintain their vigor.

In objective analysis, which is more familiar to us, phenomena such as illness, death, health, and life are treated as they actually exist in nature. We think of disease as being due to various agents, which are subject to vigorous scientific scrutiny. Thus, objective thinking is synonymous with the scientific method of problem solving. It should be pointed out, however, that humans are seldom entirely subjective or objective in attempting to explain societal or personal health problems or behavior. Most individuals tend to fall along a subjective-objective continuum, between the two extremes, as they search for explanations of illness, injury, health, or death.

Pathogenesis–the development of the disease process.

Intrapsychic–within the mind.

11

Early Ideas of Illness and Disease

The Demonic Concept

Early medicine tended to incorporate a mixture of magic and religious forces. One of the earliest ideas concerning disease was that of the demonic theory. This concept probably originated in prehistoric times and has persisted throughout history in different forms. In fact, it is still practiced in remote areas of the world and persists in some cultural groups in forms such as sorcery, witchcraft, and the "evil eye."

Basically, adherents of demonic theory thought that evil demons infected the sick individual and would devour the flesh and bones unless they could be driven out by spells, incantations, or other means. Rituals such as praying, tramping on the body, or ingesting noxious potions were usually performed by the witch doctor or native healer. If all else failed, the skull was sometimes perforated to enable the evil spirits to leave the body.

The people of early civilizations could perhaps readily accept that their life was strongly influenced by supernatural, as well as natural, forces. Thus, they could trace their misfortunes, disease, and injury to ghosts, witches, and other demonic powers. Sorceries, mystical rites, incantations, totems, and taboos reflect in part the primitive concept of the supernatural mystic. As Martin Luther in the sixteenth century so aptly stated, "pestilence, fever, and other diseases are naught else than the devil's work" (Levy-Bruhl 1936).

The Wrath of God

A second concept of disease, which resembles the demonic theory, is that disease is an expression of the wrath of an essentially righteous God animated by an innate necessity for the punishment of sin (Winslow 1980). For example, in the Old Testament numerous references are made regarding the higher concept of punishment for sin:

> If ye walk contrary unto me, and will not hearken unto me; I will bring seven times more plagues upon you according to your sins. (Leviticus 26:21)

> When ye are gathered together in your cities; I will send the pestilence among you. (Leviticus 26:25)

> So Uzziah was stricken with leprosy in punishment for his sin. (II Chronicles 26)

Even today, some people interpret illnesses such as sexually transmitted diseases and drug addiction as God's wrath for sins of impropriety.

Metaphysical Medicine

Magic is a practical means of controlling the course of life's events by a support system of laws. In a given situation, the believer feels that he or she is attaining ends by natural means, and in doing so, rationalizes decisions by what appear to be valid experimental evidence. For example, a person may state that when a rooster crows at midnight, a death in the household will occur. That person might consider employing the same kind of reasoning when relating that when a rooster is placed with hens, egg-laying will follow. Accordingly, if you relate instances in which a midnight rooster crow was not followed by a death, that person might rationalize the other situation by explaining that not all eggs are fertile (LeRiche and Milner 1971).

People can accept different methods of healing just as they accept other aspects of their cultural beliefs. Simply stated, if treatment fails, the failure can be rationalized and something else may be tried. If the patient gets well, the remedy or method of healing is generally credited with effecting the cure. If the patient dies, the remedy was not necessarily ineffective, as the patient may have been beyond help. All cultures, to some extent, have in their traditions and languages references to the biological effects of ill winds, changing seasons, the phases of the moon, and the influence of stars on behavior. Even today, some people have a strong faith in astrology—the influence of celestial bodies on human behavior and disease.

The Hippocratic Theory

Hippocrates, a Greek physician who lived from about 460 B.C. until approximately 377 B.C., was believed to be the first known individual who attributed disease to environmental factors rather than to supernatural or divine causes. For this reason, he is often referred to as the "father of epidemiology." His treatise on "Airs, Waters, and Places" was perhaps the most noteworthy of his publications and was essential to the development of a more rational approach to studying illness. Hippocrates felt that the most important aspect of medicine was to study, observe, and learn to recognize each particular disease, and to find, if possible, its cause and remedy.

In Hippocrates' time, Greek physicians believed that four properties—hot, cold, moist, and dry—operated within the universe. Each of these substances corresponded with one of the four basic humors (fluids) of the body—yellow and black bile, phlegm, and blood. Hence, health consisted of maintaining a proper balance between the humors, while disease was caused by an imbalance of the humors. Since illness was caused by the patient having either too much or too little of one or more of the basic humors, the treatment was relatively simple; the patient was bled to restore the balance. Bloodletting was often accomplished by severing a vein or by using leeches. Thus, physicians at one time were referred to as leechers.

It may seem at first that the humoral concept contributed relatively little knowledge to the field of medicine and epidemiology. Hippocrates, however, reasoned that the four humors were influenced by the presence of several innate or external factors. Advancing age, heredity, climate, humidity, wind velocity, soil, and rainfall were all believed to be capable of upsetting the balance of the humors. What is important is that Hippocrates was concerned with the relationship of humans to their physical and biological environments. He recognized that illness was not simply a random process but occurred among different populations or subgroups and also appeared to be more prevalent during different seasons of the year (Stone, O'Reilly, and Brown 1980).

The Miasmatic Theory

The miasmatic concept was another theory (prevalent during the Middle Ages) that attempted to relate environmental factors to the cause of disease. This theory held that illness was caused by certain poisonous odors, gases, or noxious wastes (miasmas), which originated in the atmosphere or from the earth and were subsequently carried by the wind to the susceptible host, who became ill after exposure. As swampy land or marshes were known to generate gas, it was logical for people to assume that malaria was caused by the presence of noxious or "bad" air. Thus, the word malaria stemmed from the Italian word *mala aria* (bad air). Actually, it was not until the end of the nineteenth century that the role of the mosquito in the spread and distribution of malaria and yellow fever provided a more rational explanation for the occurrence of these diseases. However, many current public health measures, such as the burial of the dead, garbage disposal, and sanitation reforms, originally were influenced by a belief in the miasmatic concept.

The Germ Theory

Prior to the findings reported by Robert Koch and Louis Pasteur during the latter decades of the nineteenth century, relatively little improvement was made in attempting to control and protect populations from the ravages of communicable disease. The inability to control malaria, in fact, helped to undermine the "Golden Age" of Greece between 500 and 300 B.C. Priests and lawgivers among the early Hebrews promulgated several sanitary ideas, such as isolating diseased personnel and requiring the burial of human excrement, which aided somewhat in controlling disease, as did the development of Roman baths and sewers in reducing filthborne disease. Other methods included the banishment of lepers from human society and the quarantine of incoming ships by various Mediterranean ports during the late fourteenth century in order to combat the introduction of bubonic plague (Black Death). These attempts are worth noting, but they did not really combat the spread of disease. **Epidemics** were still prevalent and were thought to be due to divine wrath, miasmas, and demonic influences.

Several individuals, however, such as Girolamo Fracastoro, John Snow, Ignas Semmelweis, Oliver Holmes, and Lemuel Shattuck, made significant contributions in their efforts to stem the tide of epidemics. Fracastoro, noted for his theory of contagion, recognized several modes of infection, by direct contact with the sick or with their garments, droppings, and the exhalations of invisible particles of breath that were discharged into the air.

Epidemic–the occurrence of disease in a region or community clearly in excess of normal expectancy.

Snow conclusively proved that cholera was a waterborne disease and also inferred that other diseases could be similarly transmitted to humans. His detailed study, using epidemiological maps of the city of London, convinced the vestrymen of St. James parish in London to remove the handle of the Broad Street pump to stop an epidemic of cholera. This action halted the distribution of contaminated drinking water, containing cholera vibrio, in the district area and abruptly halted the epidemic. We should note that Snow had no idea that cholera was caused by a microorganism, just that it had something to do with water.

Holmes, in an 1843 essay entitled "Puerperal Fever as a Private Pestilence," accused his colleagues (physicians) of carrying infection from post mortem examinations and from one patient to another on their unwashed hands. Semmelweis, in a similar vein of thought, strongly advocated that childbirth attendants (midwives and physicians) should wash their hands in a solution of chloride of lime. Deaths from **puerperal fever** were higher when physicians delivered babies. It was later discovered, when using epidemiological observations, that physicians and medical students often delivered babies without first washing their hands, even after they had dissected bodies. Thus, Semmelweis ordered his medical students to wash their hands in a lime solution before seeing any patients. Prior to this directive, the puerperal fever death rate was approximately 120 per 1,000 births. Seven months after the directive, the rate was 12 per 1,000 births (Duncan 1988).

Puerperal fever–a disease related to the period of confinement after childbirth.

Shattuck was noted for his "Report of the Sanitary Commission of Massachusetts" in 1850, which set the stage for a new era of sanitary reform in the United States. Among the many recommendations included in the report were the establishment of state and local boards of health; a system of sanitary inspectors; the collection and analysis of vital statistics; studies on the health of children; the control of alcoholism; and the inclusion of preventive medicine in medical schools.

Until the formulation of the germ theory, and even after, the idea of introducing scientific measures for the control of disease was an issue of considerable controversy within the scientific community. Many of the early contributors to the evolution of epidemiology, such as Holmes and Semmelweis, were ridiculed by their contemporaries. Also, Florence Nightingale, in 1854 during the Crimean War, found hospitals to be in a state of disarray, filth, and disorganization. Patients were often cared for by orderlies with no special training, and the English press was indignant against those responsible for their care. Nightingale attacked the problem with a staff of thirty-eight nurses, by bringing order and humanity into the care of the wounded and proving herself an able reformer and competent administrator. Even then, however, she had to battle administrative red tape in the British war office before she was able to introduce sensible sanitary reforms and measures into the nursing profession (Winslow 1980).

Louis Pasteur and Robert Koch, by virtue of their experimentation, were able to reveal the true pathogenic potential for microorganisms in disease. Soon the scientific world would turn its attention to identifying the causative agents of specific diseases. By 1857, Louis Pasteur had demonstrated the dependence of fermentation on microorganisms. Approximately seven years later, he demonstrated that the organisms causing fermentation were not generated spontaneously but came from similar microbes present in the air. Robert Koch, following the previous work of Pasteur, was able to isolate the agents responsible for tuberculosis and Asiatic cholera. Perhaps most noteworthy was his introduction of scientific rigor to proving the primary causation of disease. His postulates of a causative relation between an agent and a specific disease included the following:

1. The agent or parasite must be shown to be present in every case of the disease by isolation in a pure culture.
2. The agent must not be found in cases of other diseases.
3. The isolated agent must be capable of reproducing the disease in experimental animals.
4. The agent must be recovered from the experimental disease produced.

Today, because of more rigorous epidemiological studies of disease, we know that there are a number of errors in Koch's postulates. For instance, viruses are intracellular parasites that can multiply only within the cells of suitable hosts and cannot be cultivated in a pure culture. Also, many viruses are host specific, that is, they can infect only one host species, such as humans (for measles) or dogs (for distemper). Furthermore, infection with a particular agent does not necessarily lead to disease, as in the case of **inapparent infections.**

Inapparent infection–the presence of infection in a host without recognizable clinical signs and symptoms (same as asymptomatic infections).

Scientists such as Koch and Pasteur, and many others of the bacteriological era, made significant contributions to the evolution of epidemiology. These included the application of aseptic techniques in medicine and surgery; the development of vaccines to prevent specific diseases; the purification of water supplies; the pasteurization of milk; and the improved sanitary use of our environment.

Today, modern scientific theory dictates that there is much more to consider in the disease process besides the mere exposure of a host to a pathogenic organism. This is particularly true with respect to the chronic diseases that affect our modern society. Social, psychological, and genetic factors, which interact on the host to initiate the disease process, are studied in addition to specific microorganisms.

Models of Epidemiology

Epidemiology, broadly conceived, is concerned with the study of the determinants and distribution of health-related states or events in specified populations. In epidemiology, the major focus of study is the group rather than the individual. Epidemiology seeks to determine the distinguishing characteristics of the population that are affected by the particular illness or injury under study. Epidemiologists want to know how this population group differs from groups who do not get the disease. Thus, one can see that epidemiology is concerned with assembling and analyzing various types of information involving certain characteristics of the agent, host, and environment. In particular, epidemiology is concerned with the interaction effect of these factors between and within each other.

The Triad Model

The concept of disease causation is fundamental to epidemiology. A *cause* is usually defined as a factor whose removal leads to a reduction in the incidence of a disease or health problem. Thus, as the inadequacies of the germ theory became apparent, many epidemiologists began to formulate new theories of causation and focused their attention on the epidemiological triad of the agent, host, and environment. The triad model offered a better explanation for the dynamic interplay of the various factors in disease causation. While an agent is generally regarded as one factor that must be present for a disease to occur (as the *tubercle bacillus* must be present for tuberculosis to occur), its presence alone cannot lead to disease. That is, an agent is a **necessary factor** but not a **sufficient factor** for a disease to occur. With the triad model, however, epidemiologists began to give equal weight to the agent as a cause in disease, along with that of host and environmental factors. Recent findings from epidemiological studies do not support the exaggerated weighting given to the agent in disease causation, particularly with the knowledge gained from studying chronic diseases (Duncan 1988).

In the triad model (Figure 2.1), the host's characteristics that determine susceptibility or resistance to an agent are multiple in nature. They generally include such factors as habits, attitudes, beliefs, age, sex, race, and occupation, as well as the specific defense mechanisms contained within the host and the possible genetic influences that may operate to retard or enhance the spread of a disease. The environment itself will also act to either suppress or enhance the spread of disease. The physical characteristics of the environment, such as terrain, temperature, and precipitation, will influence the occurrence of certain diseases, such as malaria and encephalitis. In addition, the biological and social environments with which the agent and host interact will help to determine the occurrence and distribution of disease among population groups. For example, social and cultural conditions may strongly influence one's exposure and susceptibility to certain diseases, such as lung cancer. Generally lower social economic classes have higher rates of smoking and a corresponding higher incidence of lung cancer. Furthermore, some social factors may act as direct causes of disease, or may increase or decrease the probability that disease will occur in a given population.

Necessary factor–a factor, such as an agent, that is necessary for a disease to occur but whose presence alone may not be sufficient to cause disease.
Sufficient factor–an additional factor combined with the necessary factor whose presence is associated with the disease.

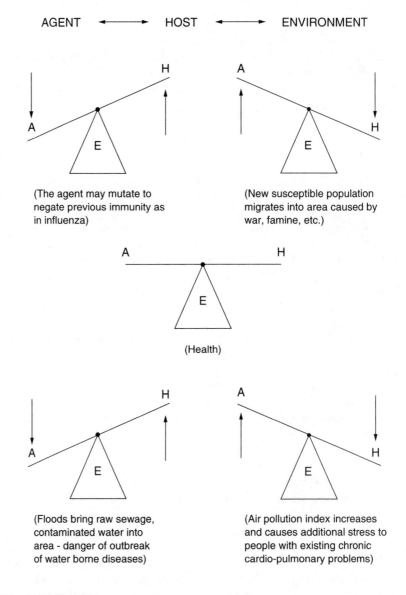

FIGURE 2.1
Agent-Host-Environment.
Modified from Fox, et. al.

AGENT ←——→ HOST ←——→ ENVIRONMENT

(The agent may mutate to negate previous immunity as in influenza)

(New susceptible population migrates into area caused by war, famine, etc.)

(Health)

(Floods bring raw sewage, contaminated water into area - danger of outbreak of water borne diseases)

(Air pollution index increases and causes additional stress to people with existing chronic cardio-pulmonary problems)

The Web Model

MacMahon and his associates developed the web model of causation to reflect the concept that multiple factors promote or inhibit the development of disease. The basic tenet underlying the web model is that "effects never depend solely on single isolated causes but develop as the result of chains of causation in which each link itself is the result of a complex genealogy of antecedents" (MacMahon and Pugh 1970). Hence, the multiplicity of antecedents creates a complex web-like structure, which may defy one's total understanding of all the variables that are related to the disease process.

Figure 2.2 illustrates the web model of causation developed by Friedman (1980) to describe the vast array of antecedents related to a myocardial infarction (heart attack). Upon examining the figure, one can observe that heredity, stress, diet, lack of exercise, smoking, and other factors can serve as antecedents to hypertension. Hypertension, in turn, is enhanced by atherosclerosis, which is characterized by a buildup of **plaque** on the interior walls of the arteries, thereby causing them to narrow, resulting in a reduced flow of blood. Hypertension in combination with atherosclerosis may result in a myocardial infarction when the blood supply to part of the heart muscle is severely reduced or stopped.

The web model can be useful to epidemiologists in identifying possible intervention points in the disease process. For example, diets low in saturated fats should help to reduce hyperlipidemia (excess fats in the blood). Physical inactivity can lead to several changes that are risk factors for heart disease. When lack of exercise is combined with overeating, excess weight and increased blood cholesterol levels can result, thereby contributing to the risk of heart disease. If physical activity and moderate eating were combined, the risk of heart disease might be lowered.

Plaque—a deposit of fatty and other substances in the inner lining of the artery (also called atheroma).

FIGURE 2.2
A Web of Causation for Myocardial Infarction.
Source: Friedman, G.D. (1980). *Primer of epidemiology*. New York: McGraw-Hill p. 4. (Reprinted with permission.)

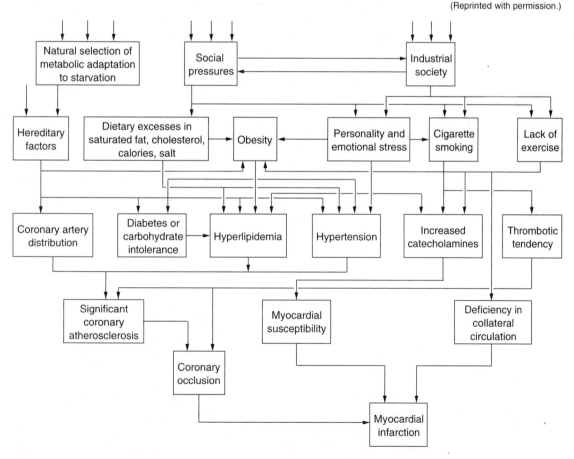

FIGURE 2.3

The Wheel Model of Man-Environment Interactions.

Source: Mausner, J. and Kramer, S. (1985). Epidemiology: An introductory text. Philadelphia: W. B. Saunders Co., pg. 36. Reprinted with permission.

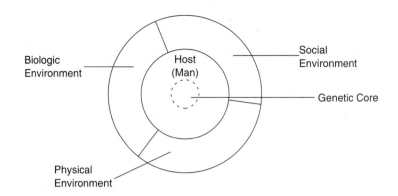

The Wheel Model

The wheel model (Figure 2.3) is another approach used by epidemiologists to describe the dynamic interplay of ecological factors (Mausner and Kramer 1985). The wheel model consists of a host and a genetic core as its main hub, with the biological, social, and physical environments serving as the outer shell. The contributions and the weight of each component would depend on the specific disease being considered. For example, in Huntington's chorea, the genetic core would assume a relatively large role, whereas in measles the genetic component would be negligible.

Similar to the web model of causation, the wheel model implies a need to identify multiple **etiological** factors of disease, without emphasizing the agent of disease (Mausner and Kramer 1985). However, the wheel model attempts to delineate the host and environment purposes of epidemiological analyses. For example, in applying the wheel model to automobile accidents, host factors would involve an analysis of age, sex, drinking habits, and personality traits. Correspondingly, the social environment might include an assessment of state and local policies regarding speed limits, sanctions, etc., whereas vehicle factors and highway designs would be incorporated into the assessment of the physical environment.

Summary

In this chapter, the authors have traced the historical foundations of disease concepts from the early origins of epidemiology to the present century, noting the contributions of many scientists involved in our quest for understanding disease causation, control, and prevention. Also, several models were introduced to show how epidemiologists try to explain the multiple factors that promote or inhibit the development of the disease process.

To understand a disease and its process, epidemiologists must investigate all the factors leading to the disease. Because of the shift in mortality from infectious disease to chronic disease in our population today, social and psychological processes are replacing specific infectious agents as causes of disease. Hence, the prevention of illness is becoming more a matter of changing the habits, customs, and life-styles of individuals. To this end, epidemiology will aid us in our attempts to identify the specific factors associated with disease and the interrelationships that affect the occurrence of disease in our modern technological society. Any change in the agent, host, or environment may upset the ecological equilibrium that had previously evolved and may enhance the occurrence and distribution of disease in a population group. For example, in the triad model, changes in the agent (a new strain of virus), the host (prolonged exposure to stress), or the environment (irrigating former arid lands for agricultural purposes and thereby providing breeding places for mosquitoes) may destroy the ecological equilibrium previously attained.

Discussion Questions

1. Briefly describe some of the early concepts of disease and their contributions to our culture and to our understanding of the disease process.
2. Why is the germ theory now considered to be inadequate for explaining the occurrence of many disease problems?
3. Describe the triad, web, and wheel models of disease. Apply an example of each model to a specific disease.
4. Describe the importance of the agent-host-environment relationship in epidemiology.
5. What are some specific uses of epidemiology in today's society?

References

Duncan, D. 1988. *Epidemiology: Basis for disease prevention and health promotion.* New York: Macmillan.

Friedman, G. D. 1980. *Primer of epidemiology.* New York: McGraw-Hill.

LeRiche, W., and J. Milner. 1971. *Epidemiology as medical ecology.* London: Churchill Livingstone.

Levi-Bruhl, L. 1936. *Primitive and the supernatural.* Trans. by L. Clare. London: Allen and Unwin.

MacMahon, B., and T. Pugh. 1970. *Epidemiologic principles and methods.* Boston: Little Brown, 1970.

Mausner, J., and S. Kramer. 1985. *Epidemiology: An introductory text.* Philadelphia: W. B. Saunders.

Stone, D., L. O'Reilly, and J. Brown. 1980. *Elementary school health education: Ecological perspectives.* Dubuque, IA: Wm. C. Brown.

Winslow, C. 1980. *The conquest of epidemic disease: A chapter in the history of ideas.* Madison, WI: University of Wisconsin Press.

CHAPTER 3

Agents of Illness

Introduction

Symptom–a phenomenon of disease or other type of illness which leads to a complaint on the part of the patient; such as the feeling of being unwell, pain, nausea, or headache.
Sign–an objective physical manifestation of disease or other type of illness, for example, high temperature or high blood pressure.

Epidemiology deals with all kinds of illnesses and health-related states or events in populations, not just disease. *Illness* is a general term meaning the feeling of being unwell, the feeling that there is something wrong with your physical or mental health. These feelings, called **symptoms** could, for example, include nausea, headache, internal pain, or depression. There may be other indications, called **signs,** that also go with illness, such as elevated temperature, bleeding from a wound, dilated pupils, or rapid pulse. These symptoms and signs are what a physician first tries to determine when a patient seeks care for an illness, and they help the physician establish a diagnosis of the complaint. A group of symptoms and signs that together distinguish a particular illness is called a *syndrome.*

It is possible for a person to feel well even when suffering from a serious disease. Many cancers and heart diseases give no feelings of illness in their early stages and will only be detected by such medical technology as a biopsy or x-ray of diseased tissue. Besides disease, other causes of illness are injuries, nutritional disorders, congenital anomalies, allergies, mental illnesses, addictions, and medical interventions (iatrogenic disorders).

Disease and Other Causes of Illness

Pathology–the science or the study of the origin, nature, and course of disease.

Disease is defined as an alteration of cells, tissues, or physiological functions that is beyond the norm. In other words, there is a recognized **pathology.** A disease has definite causes (even though we may not know what they are), a distinctive course of development, and identifiable outcomes or end results. There are two main groups of diseases: (1) *infectious* (communicable), such as influenza, malaria, or mononucleosis; and (2) *noninfectious* (chronic), such as heart disease, cancer, or stroke.

Injuries can also be classified in two groups: (1) unintentional or accidental, such as motor vehicle crashes, accidents at home, school, work, or in sports; and (2) intentional or deliberate, such as suicide, assault, rape, and homicide.

Addictions are compulsive needs for alcohol, tobacco, heroin, crack or other drugs, both legal and illegal.

Nutritional disorders include the over- or underconsumption of calories and vitamin or mineral imbalances.

Congenital anomalies are determined by the uterine environment or by genes at conception. Down's syndrome and sickle-cell anemia are two examples.

Allergies are abnormal reactions of the body to previously encountered allergens, such as pollens, grasses, dusts, or drugs.

Mental illnesses include severe forms of abnormal emotional and mental behavior, such as schizophrenia, paranoid personality, severe depression, senility, and Alzheimer's disease.

Iatrogenic disorders are diseases, injuries, allergies, or mental disorders that are caused by the practice of medicine in attempting to treat patients.

Diseases, injuries, and other causes of illness have been classified in order to standardize the reporting of the causes of death and disease. This classification is under the direction of the World Health Organization and is used by all countries in compiling death (mortality), disease, and injury (morbidity) statistics. The current *Manual of the international statistical classification of diseases, injuries and causes of death* is now in its ninth edition. An example of the classification system and its three-digit code system are given in Table 3.1.

It is important to stress that epidemiology is the scientific study of the distribution and causes of diseases, injuries, and other causes of illness with the main objective of preventing and controlling these events in populations. Medicine, on the other hand, is a professional practice to diagnose and treat all kinds of illness, with the emphasis on the individual patient. Epidemiologists use the knowledge about individuals gained in the clinical settings of medicine in order to describe and analyze illness patterns in populations. This includes the agents of illness and how they affect populations. For further discussion, see Lilienfeld and Stolley (1994) and Mausner and Kramer (1985).

Addiction–a state of being enslaved to a habit or practice or to something that is psychologically or physically habit forming, such as alcohol, tobacco, or other drugs, to the extent that cessation causes severe stress.

Agents

Disease and other forms of illness take place within the context of ecological systems, which are comprised of populations of living things and their physical, biological, and cultural environments. As we noted in Chapter 2, epidemiologists may use an ecological model with three main components (a triad) to investigate the causes of illness. The components include: the agent or agents necessary to induce a disease or other illness outcome in a person or animal; the host (persons or animals) susceptible to the agents; and the specific environment of agents and hosts that brings them into contact in time and place.

The *agents of illness* are those conditions that must be present, or absent, for disease to occur. For example, in order for the infectious disease influenza to occur, the virus of influenza must be present. The virus

TABLE 3.1 International Classification of Diseases, Injuries and Causes of Death: Selected Causes

Cause	Code
Infectious and parasitic diseases	001–139
Pertussis	033
Measles	055
Malignant neoplasms	140–208
Cancer of the stomach	151
Cancer of the lung	162
Diabetes mellitus	250
Nutritional deficiencies	260–269
Major cardiovascular diseases	390–448
Ischemic heart disease	410–414
Acute myocardial infarction	410
Atherosclerosis	440
Appendicitis	540–543
Chronic liver disease and cirrhosis	571
Complications of pregnancy, childbirth, and the puerperium	630–676
Congenital anomalies	740–759
Accidents and adverse effects	E800–E949
Motor vehicle	E810–E825
Suicide	E950–E959
Homicide	E960–E978

Source: From World Health Organization. 1975. *Manual of the international statistical classification of disease, injuries and causes of death*, 9th rev. Geneva, Switzerland: WHO.

in this case is the necessary agent. Illness may also result from the lack of an agent, as, for example, in nutritional deficiency. For some diseases there may be several necessary agents, each acting in particular ways. Certain cancers, for instance, require specific chemical agents acting as promoters of tumors and others acting as initiators to trigger the disease. In other situations, several different agents may produce the same end result—any one is sufficient to cause illness. For example, fists, knives, and handguns are all agents of energy sufficient to cause homicide. Some agents may cause some proportion of one or more diseases, as is the case with tobacco smoke, which is a contributing agent for heart disease, emphysema, and cancers of the larynx, esophagus, and lung.

Classification of Agents

Agents can be classified into six groups:

1. *Infectious agents* (viruses, rickettsia, bacteria, fungi, protozoa, and helminths) cause infectious diseases.

Agents of Illness

2. *Chemical agents* that are ingested through the mouth, inhaled through the nose or mouth, or absorbed through the skin can cause noninfectious diseases (such as heart disease and cancers), allergies, nutritional disorders, and injuries. Chemical agents also include poisons from snake bites, poisonous plants, and industrial chemicals.
3. *Physical agents* include excessive heat, electricity, radiation, sharp instruments, bullets, falling and crushing, animal bites, natural disasters, or drowning.
4. *Psychological agents* are mental and physical stressors (for example, excessive noise, overcrowding, oppressions, physical diseases, pain, and addictions).
5. *Social agents* are underlying causes of illnesses, for example, poverty, unemployment, homelessness, war, peer pressures, unsafe technologies, persecutions, and social violence.
6. *Genetic agents* are hereditary factors that cause genetic disorders or make individuals susceptible to other illness-causing agents.

All agents may act singly or in combination. For example, every episode of infectious disease in a person is a combination of physical and psychological agents, because the illness has an emotional effect.

Agent-Host-Environment Interactions

The *host* is the person or animal who has the illness, which is a consequence of being exposed to and affected by the agents in a suitable environment. Remember that illness in its various forms occurs in individual human beings or animals. In this sense, it is a physiological and psychological phenomenon. Illness is also a characteristic of groups of people or populations. In this sense, it is a biopsychosocial phenomenon. This distinction is important when we study the causes of disease and other forms of illness, because we need to understand the processes at both the individual and population level.

Not everyone is a host to every form of illness. Hosts are those individuals who come into contact with the agent and who are susceptible to it. A susceptible host, in the case of a virus for an infectious disease, would be a person not having sufficient resistance to prevent infection. A person who has been immunized against a particular infectious agent, such as tetanus, is much less susceptible to infection from that agent. We are all susceptible to some agents, for example, injury from high doses of nuclear radiation.

The *environment* is the surroundings of the host that provide appropriate conditions for the agent and the host to interact to produce illness. Except for genetic agents that originate at conception, all agents arise from the environment of the host. For the unborn child, the environment is the mother's womb. Our most intimate common contacts with the environment are through air, food, water, and skin contact. For human beings, the environment is always a combination of physical, biological, and cultural conditions.

Disease and other forms of illness can be viewed as an outcome of the interactions between agent, host, and environment, which are functioning as an ecological system. For each specific illness, there is a particular ecological system with characteristic agent, host, and environment interactions. Two examples of these interactions, one for an infectious disease and one for a noninfectious disease, are given in Table 3.2. Note that each disease has an element of time (called the **incubation period** in infectious diseases and the *latent period* in noninfectious diseases), which is the period between initial exposure to an agent with susceptible host response and the appearance of the first sign or symptom of the illness in question. This period of time can vary from a few hours, in the case of some infectious diseases, to many decades, in the case of some noninfectious diseases.

Epidemiologists search for the causes of illness within the context of this ecological system of agent-host-environment. Because it is a system, all components interact with and affect one another, and all are important, either directly or indirectly, in causing the outcome of the illness. For any episode of illness in an individual, there will be immediate physiological and psychological causes, but there are also likely to be underlying biological, physical, and cultural causes as well.

In Table 3.3 two causes of death, suicide and cancer of the stomach, are given as examples. The immediate cause of death in the suicide is drowning, a type of asphyxia related to either the aspiration of fluid or the obstruction of the airway caused by larynx spasm while in the water. Death occurs due to lack of oxygen. Underlying the drowning, however, was the intentional act on the part of the host to commit suicide. This, in turn, was due to mental depression, and, successively, to being homeless,

---

TABLE 3.2 Examples of Agent-Host-Environment Interactions

Disease	Agent	Host	Environment
Noninfectious: mesothelioma (cancer of the chest lining) Latent period: median 35 years.	Asbestos	10 percent of workers routinely exposed to asbestos fibers; chance exposure by others	Worksites using asbestos and places where asbestos fibers become airborne, as in the demolition of old buildings
Infectious: acquired immunodeficiency syndrome (AIDS) Incubation period: median 9 years.	Human immunodeficiency virus	Susceptible persons exposed to virus through sexual activity, contaminated blood products, shared needles, or as fetus or newborns	Bodily fluids (semen, blood); cultural practices of sexual behavior and drug use; medical services with contaminated blood supplies

Source: Authors

TABLE 3.3 Examples of Immediate and Underlying Causes of Illness

Causes	Suicide	Cancer of the stomach
1. Immediate	Drowning	Pneumonia
2. Underlying	Suicide*	Secondary cancers of the liver and lung
3. Underlying	Depression	Cancer of the stomach*
4. Underlying	Homeless	Chronic gastritis
5. Underlying	Unwanted pregnancy	Nitrosamines?
6. Underlying	No access to social supports	Diet rich in salt and poor fresh fruits and vegetables?

Source: Authors

Note: Items 1, 2, and 3 would be recorded on death certificates.

*These entries would be recorded in official statistics as the cause of death.

having an unwanted pregnancy, and not having access to social supports that might have altered the course of events.

In the case of cancer of the stomach, the immediate cause of death was pneumonia, a severe inflammation and congestion of the lungs causing death by asphyxiation. The underlying causes, in succession, were: secondary cancers of the lung and liver, which were metastases (transplants) from a primary cancer of the stomach; a history of chronic gastritis, probably initiated by carcinogens in the diet (nitrosamines are suspected) and promoted by a diet rich in salt (which helps expose the stomach tissue directly to stomach contents); and a diet poor in fresh fruits and vegetables, which are believed to have a protective effect against stomach cancer. In any epidemiological investigation of the causes of disease and other forms of illness, immediate and underlying causes are all important. In general, the more we understand about the underlying causes, the more effectively we can prevent and control illness.

The concept of immediate and underlying causes is recognized on official death certificates, where one immediate and up to two underlying causes may be recorded. For official statistics, only one cause is selected. This is the cause believed to carry the best explanation for the event. In the examples in Table 3.3, the official statistics would list "suicide" and "cancer of the stomach," respectively. This topic is taken up again in Chapter 6.

Infectious Diseases

An *infectious disease* is a clinically apparent disease in humans or animals resulting from an infection. *Clinically apparent* means that the disease can be detected by clinical symptoms and signs. *Infection* is the entry and establishment of an infectious agent in the body, the agent being a virus, rickettsia, bacteria, fungi, protozoa, or helminths. Infection is not the same as infectious disease, and most infections do not cause infectious diseases—the hosts feel fine, and the infections cannot be detected by any clinical signs. These *inapparent infections* are also called *subclinical* or *asymptomatic*.

Some infectious agents can infect only humans, so we are the only hosts or populations at risk. Examples of diseases caused by such agents are measles, mumps, and poliomyelitis. Other infectious agents are common to humans as well as other vertebrate animal species and can move from one species to another. There is thus more than one set of hosts, or *reservoirs*, of infection. Diseases caused by these agents are called **zoonoses** or zoonotic diseases and include, for example, rabies, typhus fever, and tetanus. Table 3.4 lists the major infectious diseases, the agents that cause them, and whether they are zoonotic.

Zoonoses–an infection or infectious disease of vertebrate animals that may be transmitted under natural conditions to human beings.

In order for an infection to take place, an infectious agent has to gain entrance to the cells and tissues of the host where it can find its habitat. The correct portal of entry is important. The influenza virus must find its way into the respiratory system via the mouth and nasal passages; tetanus spores enter muscle tissue via deep wounds. The infectious agent then has to adapt to the host's tissues and immunological system and multiply. It is possible that the host's defenses might sufficiently react to overcome the infection at an early stage. Then the infectious agent has to have an effective portal of exit from the host (which is often but not always the same portal as entry), and it has to have a mechanism of transmission to a new host in order to maintain its life cycle.

Biological Characteristics of Agents

Infectious agents have complex biological characteristics that can be important in the prevention and control of disease. For instance, one characteristic is whether the agent is single or multiple in type, and whether it has more than one serotype or subtype. The measles virus is a single type of agent, but infectious hepatitis is caused by five known types, each with distinctive epidemiological characteristics. The human immunodeficiency virus that causes AIDS has two serologically different types (HIV-1 and HIV-2) but with similar epidemiological characteristics. Influenza has three main types of virus, but each type has several strains. The influenza virus is also capable of developing new strains at irregular intervals, a process called *genetic shifting*. The control of a disease is simplified if it is caused by a single agent, but control becomes increasingly complex when there are multiple and shifting agents.

Transmission–the transfer of an agent from one person to another, or the spread of an agent through the environment by direct contact, or, indirectly, by vehicle, vector, or airborne mechanism.

Transmission of Agents to Hosts

After an agent exits its natural reservoir, or habitat, it may be transmitted to a susceptible host in several ways. These modes of transmission are classified as either direct (via direct contact and droplet spread) or indirect (via airborne, vehicleborne, and vectorborne—including mechanical and biological—**transmission**). In *direct transmission*, there is an immediate transfer of the agent from a reservoir to a susceptible host by direct

TABLE 3.4 Agents for Major Infectious Diseases

Virus

Acquired immunodeficiency syndrome
  (AIDS)
Arthropod-borne Viral Fevers*
Chickenpox
Common cold
Hepatitis A, B, C, Delta, E
Herpes simplex
Influenza
Measles
Mononucleosis
Mumps
Poliomyelitis
Rabies*
Rubella
Viral gastroenteritis
Warts

Rickettsia

Q fever*
Rickettsial fevers (tick-borne)*
Rickettsialpox*
Scrub typhus*
Typhus, endemic (flea-borne)*
Typhus, epidemic (louse-borne)*

Chlamydia

Lymphogranuloma venereum
Psittacosis*
Trachoma

Bacteria

Anthrax*
Botulism
Brucellosis*
Cholera
Diphtheria
Gonorrhea
Legionellosis
Leprosy
Listeriosis*
Pertussis
Plague*
Salmonellosis*
Shigellosis
Staphylococcal disease
Streptococcal disease
Tetanus*
Tuberculosis*
Tularemia*
Typhoid fever

Spirochete

Leptospirosis*
Lyme disease*
Pinta
Relapsing fever*
Syphilis
Yaws

Mycota (Fungi)

Aspergillosis
Blastomycosis
Candidiasis
Coccidioidomycosis*
Histoplasmosis*

Protozoa

Amebiasis
Giardiasis
Leishmaniasis*
Malaria*
Toxoplasmosis*
Trypanosomiasis, African*
Trypanosomiasis, American*

Helminth

Angiostrongyliasis*
Ascariasis*
Echinococcosis*
Filariasis
Hookworm disease*
Onchocerciasis*
Schistosomiasis*
Stronglyoidiasis*
Taeniasis*
Trichinosis*
Trichuriasis*

Multiple

Conjunctivitis
Diarrhea
Foodborne intoxication
Meningitis
Pneumonia
Rat-bite fever*

Source: From Benenson, A. S., ed. 1990. *Control of communicable diseases in man*, 15th ed.
Washington D.C.: American Public Health Association.

*Indicates zoonotic disease.

Droplet nuclei–dried residue of droplets that congeal and can be suspended in air currents.

Vector–an arthropod insect that transmits an infectious agent either biologically, through its internal organism, or mechanically, by conveying infectious agents on its legs or through the gastrointestinal tract.

Vehicle–an inanimate object, such as drinking water, food, bedding, or a toy, that transmits an infectious agent because it has been contaminated.

Carrier–a person or animal who harbors a specific infectious agent without having evidence of clinical disease and who can serve as a potential source of infection.

contact or droplet spread. *Reservoirs* are generally defined as the living organisms or inanimate matter (i.e., soil) in which the infectious agent lives and multiplies. Thus, reservoirs of infection include humans, animals, and environmental sources.

Direct contact occurs through kissing, skin-to-skin contact, and sexual intercourse. Direct contact also refers to contact with soil or vegetation harboring infectious organisms. Thus, infectious mononucleosis ("kissing disease") and gonorrhea are spread from person to person by direct contact. Hookworm is spread by direct contact with contaminated soil. *Droplet spread* refers to spray with relatively large, short-range aerosols, which can be produced by sneezing, coughing, or even talking. Droplet spread is classified as direct because the transmission is by direct spray over a few feet, before the droplets fall to the ground.

In *indirect transmission*, an agent is carried from a reservoir to a susceptible host by suspended air particles, **droplet nuclei,** or by animate **(vector)** or inanimate **(vehicle)** intermediaries. Most vectors are arthropods such as mosquitoes, fleas, and ticks. These may carry the agent through purely mechanical means. For example, flies carry shigella on their appendages; fleas carry Yersinia pestis (the agent that causes plague) in the gut and deposit the agent on the skin of a new host. In mechanical transmission, the agent does not multiply or undergo physiological changes in the vector. This is in contrast to instances in which an agent undergoes part of its life cycle inside a vector before being transmitted to a new host. When the agent undergoes changes within the vector, the vector is serving both as an intermediate host and as a mode of transmission. This type of indirect transmission is a *biological transmission.* For example, Guinea worm disease and many other vectorborne diseases have complex life cycles that require an intermediate host. Since the agent undergoes part of its life cycle in the intermediate host, the agent cannot be transmitted by the intermediate host until the agent has completed that part of its life cycle. Therefore, this is an indirect, vectorborne, biological transmission (Centers for Disease Control 1992).

Some agents can exist for long periods of time in a host without causing a clinical disease, and yet they can still be capable of infecting others. This is called a carrier state, in which a host is a **carrier** for a particular infectious disease. Typhoid fever and hepatitis type B have a carrier state.

As we noted earlier, there is a time interval between the first contact with an infectious agent and the appearance of the first sign or symptom of a disease. This interval is called the **incubation period**, and it varies considerably, depending on the infectious disease. The incubation period for influenza, for example, is 24–72 hours; for measles it is 8–13 days; and for AIDS 3–12 years. Each infectious disease also has a **period of communicability**, during which the agent is capable of being transmitted from one host to another. The period of communicability for influenza is 3 days; for measles it is about 5 days; and for AIDS it is unknown.

Some infectious diseases are prevalent all year round. These diseases are usually confined to human hosts and are transmitted by direct contact. They include the common cold, sexually transmitted diseases, and the common diseases of childhood, such as measles, mumps, and chickenpox. Some infectious diseases are distinctly seasonal, and these are usually zoonotic diseases, in which animal hosts or insect vectors are more active in one season than in another. Lyme disease is one example, and other diseases would involve cases where human hosts are exposed to infectious agents because of seasonal activities, such as hunters who are exposed to game that is infected with tularemia.

Immunity

Exposure to infectious agents and the likelihood of developing disease differ greatly between hosts. Infection results in an immunological response by the host whereby antibodies are normally produced to resist and overcome the infection. While some individuals can resist infections better than others, any experience with a particular infectious agent usually leaves the host with some measure of specific immunity to future infections from the same agent.

Immunity is classified as being *active* if the host produces its own antibodies, and *passive* if the host possesses antibodies but is not capable of producing its own. Immunity is also classified as being *natural* if it derives from infection and recovery, and as *artificial* if it is the result of vaccination. Thus, active natural immunity is acquired through infection and recovery. Once a person has had chicken pox, for instance, that person generally is immune for life. Most infectious diseases leave the host with some measure of natural active immunity to subsequent infections by the same agent, but some diseases leave very little immunity. For some diseases, active artificial immunity may be obtained through vaccination. Some vaccines are very effective, such as the one for tetanus; others are weak, such as the one for typhoid fever, which serves to reduce the severity of the disease and the risk of death. Passive natural immunity is possessed by newborn infants for the first few months of life, because they have shared the bloodstream of their mother in the fetus, which contained whatever antibodies she had developed to specific infectious diseases. Passive artificial immunity can be obtained by injecting antibodies from a person or animal who is actively immune to one who is not. For example, gamma globulin, the antibody fraction of blood plasma, is injected to give short-term protection against infectious hepatitis and measles.

Infectious Disease Control

All of the factors we have just reviewed are important to epidemiologists as they consider the options for the prevention and control of infectious diseases. Despite the remarkable successes of the last 100 years, however, only one infectious disease has been eradicated. This is smallpox, which was declared eradicated by the World Health Organization in 1980. The

Period of communicability–the time or times during which an infectious agent may be transmitted directly or indirectly from one infected person to another, or from an infected animal to a person, or from an infected person to an animal (including insects).

Immunity–protection from, or being susceptible to, a particular disease. This is usually associated with the presence of antibodies or cells in the host that have a specific action on the infectious agent causing the disease.

eradication of smallpox was possible for the following reasons (Evans 1985):

1. Smallpox was a single virus with no subtypes.
2. The virus was confined to human hosts.
3. It was transmitted by direct contact only.
4. There was no carrier state.
5. It produced an unmistakable clinical disease easily diagnosed by anyone, and there were no inapparent subclinical cases.
6. It had a short incubation period of 7–17 days and a period of communicability of about 3 weeks.
7. Following recovery, immunity was permanent, with distinctive facial scars to allow the easy identification of all cases.
8. For smallpox there is a highly effective thermostable vaccine, meaning that it can be used in communities that do not have electricity for refrigeration.
9. The disease has a distinct seasonality, so there was a greater opportunity for organizing control measures.
10. When the World Health Organization began to plan the eradication of smallpox, finances were available and the political and social climate for action was favorable.
11. Smallpox was a hated disease that everyone agreed should be eliminated.

With smallpox, control teams were able to isolate the disease reservoirs to particular populations and, with mass community vaccinations, to reduce the pools of infection to levels where the virus could not survive. Because there were no other species involved, no subclinical cases, and no carrier states, the task was greatly simplified. The smallpox virus was apparently not capable of developing new strains, and the vaccine gave immunity for several years. The fact that the disease and the vaccination left distinctive permanent scars made it easy to identify nonimmune, susceptible persons. Also, the thermostable vaccine could be taken quickly to remote, poor communities anywhere in the world.

There is no other human infectious disease that has the same characteristics as smallpox. Measles and poliomyelitis can be controlled in regions where vigorous vaccination programs are maintained, but worldwide eradication is unlikely because of technical, economic, and political constraints. The best hope for the control of most infectious diseases is prevention through the discovery of effective vaccines, or achieving some degree of control, as with the elimination of malaria from some parts of the world through control of its mosquito vector. AIDS is proving to be difficult to control because it has a genetically shifting virus, a large unknown pool of subclinical cases, an incubation period lasting from three to twelve years, no vaccine, and an adverse social and political climate. Because the human immunodeficiency virus that causes AIDS is primarily transmitted by sexual intercourse and involves the culture of sexual behavior, it is especially difficult to intervene in the disease cycle.

The effort is further complicated by societal values that discourage sex education in schools and open discussion of the interaction of sexual behavior and the disease.

Noninfectious Diseases

Noninfectious diseases cause nonreversible pathological alterations. In other words, they cause permanent physical damage to the host, and most cases require special rehabilitation or long-term care. Noninfectious diseases include the major causes of death in most industrialized societies—heart disease, cancers, and stroke—and many other causes of death and disability, such as diabetes, ulcers, hernias, arthritis, varicose veins, gout, and osteoporosis. We usually associate noninfectious diseases with the organ or body part that is affected, such as lung cancer, coronary artery disease, and cirrhosis of the liver. Unlike infectious diseases, there are rarely single agents that lead to a disease. Instead, there are usually several agents that singly, or in combination, can produce the same noninfectious disease. For example, cigarette smoke is a major contributing causal agent for diseases of the heart, lung cancer, and emphysema. It does not, however, cause all the cases of these diseases; and not everyone who smokes will die of these diseases. Not everyone is susceptible to a particular noninfectious disease, for physiological, psychological, or genetic reasons. For most noninfectious diseases, we know much more about the pathology and end results than we do about the causes or process of the disease. Most heart disease, cancers, and stroke take twenty to forty years to develop and may be the result of a lifetime of particular dietary patterns or using drugs such as tobacco and alcohol.

Risk Factors

Epidemiological research has identified certain risk factors that are associated with some noninfectious diseases. A *risk factor* is an environmental or behavioral factor that is associated with increasing the risk of a particular illness or of a cause of death. For example, hypertension is a risk factor for ischemic heart disease; increasing age is a risk factor for cancers of the colon and lung. Risk factors are associated with an illness and are not necessarily causal factors. A *causal factor* is one that has been established beyond reasonable doubt as a causal agent of an illness.

Information about risk factors can be used to prevent or control disease by educating people to change their habits; by reducing the exposure to risk factors; and by developing policies to modify the environment, such as introducing food additives to protect against bacterial growth, reducing salt in commercial foods, and eliminating occupational exposures to toxic chemicals. For instance, risk factors for coronary heart disease include diets rich in saturated fats, cigarette smoking, obesity, and hypertension; a risk factor for lung cancer is cigarette smoking; and for stroke, a risk factor is hypertension. Exposure to carcinogenic chemicals in industrial occupations poses the risk of cancers of the liver, brain, bladder, lung, and skin. For many noninfectious diseases, no risk factors have yet been identified. For all of them, though, the causes are believed to be a combination of primarily environmental factors and, to a lesser degree, biological factors that condition the physiological, psychological, and genetic susceptibility of individuals.

Injuries and Their Control

Injuries are the leading cause of death and disability among children and young adults in industrialized countries and in most less-industrialized countries as well. In the United States, injuries kill more people aged one through thirty-four than all diseases combined, and they are the leading cause of death up to age forty-four (National Research Council 1985).

An injury is caused by an acute exposure to energy, such as heat, electricity, a car crash, a fall, or a bullet. It may also be caused by a sudden loss of energy, such as the loss of oxygen when drowning. As we mentioned previously, injuries may be categorized as unintentional or intentional. The major categories of injury deaths in the United States are motor vehicle crashes, firearms, falls and jumps, drownings, and poisonings, in that order.

There are three major strategies for injury prevention and control:

1. *Persuade* persons at risk of injury to alter their behavior for increased self-protection, for example, to fasten car seat belts, use crash helmets on motorcycles, use smoke detectors, and avoid walking alone at night in risky environments.
2. *Require* individual behavior change by law, such as laws to require the use of seat belts, to control alcohol use, to use safety equipment on the job, and to prohibit the use of dangerous chemicals or weapons.
3. *Provide* automatic protection by product and environmental design, for example, airbags and automatic seat belts in cars, highway overpasses over railroads, safe industrial processes in factories, and automatic sprinkler systems in buildings.

In general, unintentional injuries are easier to prevent or to control than intentional injuries, because they rarely involve complex social or behavioral situations and more is known about their causes and patterns of occurrence. For example, rape, which is a brutal, intentional crime of violence, has proven very difficult to prevent. It is estimated that one million rapes are committed each year in the United States, almost all by men against women. Rape is a violent form of physical and psychological injury and is not primarily a sexual act, whether it occurs between strangers, acquaintances, or intimates. It has life-shattering consequences for victims and disruptive effects for society. What is known about rape?

1. Most rapes are committed by male acquaintances of females.
2. Most rapes take place inside homes and usually in bedrooms.
3. Overindulgence in alcoholic drinks is associated with most rapes.
4. Rape is rarely committed by a psychotic person. It is a criminal expression of power and domination.
5. Sexual violence may be linked to various sources, such as the mass media, pornography, childhood experiences, and family violence.
6. Sex-role stereotypes "make it permissible" for men to dominate women, to use violence rather than communication, and to not respect a woman's right to say no to sex or assault.

Epidemiologists work toward preventing and controlling rape as well as all kinds of injuries. They try to better describe the incidence and patterns of occurrence of injuries (in terms of time, place, and persons) and to investigate their immediate and underlying causes. In the case of rape we need to replace ignorance and myth with information and understanding. We also have to learn why some men behave so brutally toward women, why some women cannot speak out about their attackers, and what the role of alcohol is in the cause of rape (U.S. Public Health Service 1986).

The Natural History and Spectrum of Disease

The natural history of a disease refers to the progress of a disease in an individual over time, in the absence of intervention. The process begins with the exposure to or accumulation of factors capable of causing the disease. Without medical intervention, the process ends with recovery, disability, or death. The stages in the natural history of a disease are shown in Figure 3.1. Most diseases have a characteristic natural history (which is poorly understood for many diseases), although the time frame and specific manifestations of a disease may vary from person to person. With a particular individual, the usual course of a disease may be halted at any point in the progression by preventive and therapeutic measures, host factors, and other influences.

The spectrum of disease is the sequence of events, or natural history, that occurs in a human being from the time of exposure to the causal agent until death. The spectrum concept is especially useful for studying infectious and noninfectious diseases when each disease has a distinctive course of events over time, assuming that there are no treatments to interrupt the natural history. Of course, in practice, most illnesses end in recovery, either because the attack was mild for the host or treatment was successful. With some forms of illness, such as severe injuries, the time

FIGURE 3.1
Natural History of
Disease.

Source: Principles of Epi-
demiology. Atlanta GA. U.S.
Department of Health and
Human Services. Centers
for Disease Control and
Prevention, 1992, p. 43.

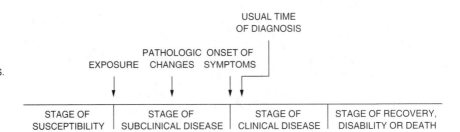

between exposure to the agent and death may be very short. In such cases, a spectrum of disease has little utility.

In infectious diseases (as shown in Figure 3.1), the spectrum begins when the host is exposed to the infectious agent. This leads to the first stage of susceptibility, in which the factors necessary for infection and the disease process are in place. Once infection is established, the second stage of the process is subclinical disease or inapparent infection. There are pathological changes during this stage, but no signs or symptoms are detectable. The third stage is clinical disease, in which the disease can be detected by signs or symptoms. The disease progresses from mild to severe effects on the host, and the spectrum ends in death.

In noninfectious diseases, the spectrum follows a similar progression from initial exposure to a causal agent, through subclinical and clinical disease, to death. Most cancers pass through three stages: **dysplasia, cancer in situ,** and invasive cancer. Cerebrovascular disease (stroke) passes through the stages of atherosclerosis in cerebral arteries, mild transient disruptions of blood supply to the brain, and stroke (a sudden major disruption of blood supply to the brain).

The spectrum of disease is a useful concept within which to examine different approaches to prevention and control. If the entire spectrum for a particular disease is well understood, there may be several options at various stages for interventions that could prevent or control severe disease outcomes. For most infectious and noninfectious diseases, we know very little about the subclinical stages. In some infectious diseases, such as poliomyelitis, over 90 percent of the infections are subclinical, meaning that only the "tip of the iceberg" is observable as clinical disease. This vast reservoir of subclinical infection allows the virus to be transmitted from host to host without human awareness. This is one reason why poliomyelitis would be very difficult to eradicate. Measles, on the other hand, is a disease in which over 90 percent of the infections lead to clinical disease, making it much more obvious and easier to control.

Dysplasia–an
abnormal
development in cells
that may be
precancerous and
may lead to the
development of
cancer cells.

Cancer in situ–an
early stage of cancer
in which the tumor is
still confined to the
cells of origin.

Summary

Agents of illness are those factors or conditions that by their presence, or absence, are necessary to cause illness. The mere presence of an agent is not sufficient to cause illness; the interactions of other components of the ecological system of agent-host-environment will affect whether or not illness will occur. There are many forms of illness: disease, injuries, additions, nutritional disorders, congenital anomalies, allergies, mental illness, and iatrogenic disorders. The agents of illness can be classified as infectious, chemical, physical, psychological, social, or genetic. Together with susceptible hosts and suitable environments, agents act alone or in combination to cause illness. The causes of illness may be immediate or underlying. The prevention and control of an illness are based on the knowledge of its biological and social causes, its natural history, and its distribution in populations.

A clinically apparent disease can be detected by clinical signs and symptoms. However, many infections do not result in clinical cases and are categorized as asymptomatic. For infection to occur, the infectious organism must gain entry into a susceptible host, multiply, have an appropriate portal of exit and be transmitted to a new susceptible host.

Immunity to a specific disease may be classified as active or passive or natural or artificial depending on the manner in which it was acquired.

Noninfectious diseases include a variety of conditions such as heart disease, diabetes, gout, cancer, etc., in which a variety of agents acting either by themselves or in combination with others produce a given disease. In an attempt to more adequately understand the nature of noninfectious diseases, epidemiologists have attempted to study risk factors that may be associated with a given disease.

In order to more fully assess injuries and their control, epidemiologists have employed three major strategies; persuasion, requiring behavior change through legal mechanisms, and providing protection through product and environmental design.

Finally, the natural history and spectrum of disease is discussed with reference to different approaches to disease prevention and control.

Discussion Questions

1. For each of the following, identify the likely agent or agents, host, and environment: (a) measles, (b) motor-vehicle crash, (c) addiction to alcohol.
2. What are the main causes of illness?
3. What are the main categories of agents that cause illness?
4. Distinguish between the immediate and underlying causes of injuries in a car-train accident in which the car's driver was intoxicated.
5. Describe what a risk factor is and present several examples. How can knowledge of a risk factor be used in public health programs?
6. Discuss the major strategies used in injury prevention and control.

References

Benenson, A. S., ed. 1990. *Control of communicable diseases in man*, 15th ed. Washington D.C.: American Public Health Association.

Centers for Disease Control. 1992. *Principles of epidemiology*. Atlanta, GA: U.S. Department of Health and Human Services.

Evans, A. S. 1985. The eradication of communicable disease: Myth or reality? *American Journal of Epidemiology* 122:197–207.

Lilienfeld, D. E. and P. D. Stolley. 1994. *Foundations of epidemiology*, 3rd ed. New York: Oxford University Press.

Mausner, J. S. and S. Kramer. 1985. *Epidemiology*, 2nd ed. Philadelphia: W. B. Saunders.

National Research Council and the Institute of Medicine. 1985. *Injury in America*. Washington, D.C.: National Academy Press.

U.S. Public Health Service. 1986. Surgeon General's Workshop on Violence and Public Health Report. Washington, D.C.: Government Printing Office.

World Health Organization. 1975. *Manual of the international statistical classification of disease, injuries, and causes of death*. 9th rev. Geneva, Switzerland: WHO.

CHAPTER 4

Host Factors and Their Influence on Disease and Health

Introduction

Inherent differences in certain attributes of the host may significantly contribute to one's susceptibility or resistance to disease. In addition, there are agent and environmental factors that may influence the frequency of occurrence or severity of the disease process. As we have noted earlier, the modern approach to studying disease is based on studying the interaction of the host, the causative agent, and the environment. This chapter will focus primarily on the host and host-agent interactions in infectious diseases. Chapter 7 will elaborate further on descriptive epidemiology, which involves detailed descriptions of personal attributes, place, and time patterns as they relate to epidemiological investigations.

Characteristics of the host generally include age, sex, ethnic group, socioeconomic status, marital status, previous disease, life-style, heredity, and nutrition. All of these attributes are important to the extent that they affect the risk of exposure to a disease agent, the host's resistance to susceptibility to infection, and the final outcome of a specific disease.

Analyzing the Influence of Host Factors

Host factors are generally characteristics of subgroups of a certain population that may influence the frequency of occurrence or severity of a disease process. It is important to note the following information concerning host factors:

1. All possible host factors are not pertinent to every disease.
2. Each host factor may interact with other host factors or with factors associated with the agent or the environment.
3. Host factors are dynamic, and their relative importance in any specific disease situation may vary in magnitude.
4. Even when the presence of a specific host factor and the disease can be demonstrated to be statistically significant, this aspect alone does not guarantee that the factor is a determinant of the disease.

Consequently, the first step for epidemiologists is to determine the importance of a host factor in the occurrence of a disease. They must resolve the following question: Is the association between the presence of the factor and the occurrence of the disease strong enough to be considered statistically significant?

Two-By-Two Tables

Statistical evaluation depends on the nature of the data under study. For example, with attribute data (i.e., "either-or" data, such as male/female, disease/non-disease, exposure to the suspect factor/no exposure), a two-by-two table can be constructed and a chi-square test applied to determine the significance of the association.

Epidemiologists use two-by-two tables to study the association between an exposure and disease. These tables are convenient for comparing persons with and without the exposure, and those with and without the disease. Table 4.1 shows the generic format of such a table. The letters a, b, c, and d within the four cells of the two-by-two table refer to the number of persons with the disease status indicated to its left. For example, c represents the number of persons in the study who have the disease but who were not exposed to the factor being studied.

Let us now look at Table 4.2. From the data in that two-by-two table, one can determine the actual or estimated risk of tuberculosis for alcoholics and nondrinkers by applying the appropriate calculations for **relative** and **attributable risk,** which will be discussed in further detail in

TABLE 4.1 Two-by-Two Table

	Disease present (D)	Disease absent ($\bar{D}$)	
Factor present (F)	a	b	a + b
Factor absent ($\bar{F}$)	c	d	c + d
	a + c	b + d	a + b + c + d

Source: Authors

TABLE 4.2 A Comparison of Persons with Tuberculosis by Presence of Alcoholism

	Persons with TB	Persons without TB	Total
Alcoholics	38	12	50
Nondrinkers	8	92	100
Total	46	104	150

Source: Authors

Host Factors and Their Influence on Disease and Health

Chapter 8. Also, a chi-square test $(X)^2$ may be employed to estimate the likelihood that some factor other than chance accounts for the apparent relationship between alcoholism and tuberculosis (Roht et al. 1982).

Attack Rates

When epidemiologists study acute infectious disease, especially epidemics, the association between a host factor and the occurrence of an illness is often described by calculating *attack rates*. This term is defined as follows:

$$\text{Attack rate for factor } A = \frac{\text{Number of persons who possess factor } A \text{ and became ill}}{\text{Total number of persons who possess factor } A \text{ and were considered } at\ risk} \times 100$$

This use of the term *rate* is technically incorrect, since the *velocity* of disease occurrence is not being measured. What is being measured is the probability of illness among those who possess factor A. Note that the degree to which the presence of factor A is associated with the occurrence of the disease can only be evaluated by contrast. In this instance, the contrast is between the probability of illness for those with factor A versus the probability of illness for those without factor A. Attack rates are commonly used in disease outbreaks associated with the consumption of contaminated foods, in order to identify the food most likely to have been responsible.

Age—An Important Host Factor

Of all the host factors, age is the most important, for no disease process occurs with the same frequency at all ages (Mausner and Kramer 1985). This is especially obvious when one considers the relationship of age to the following biological phenomena, which are critical to the science of epidemiology.

1. Risk of exposure to a specific disease agent. With household contacts, especially, there is a greater risk of exposure to infected cases or carriers. The longer one is around, the more likely it is that one will contract something.
2. Duration of exposure. This is particularly important to the cumulative effect of environmental agents, and to those diseases requiring a prolonged incubation period, e.g., the slow viral infections and perhaps the **neoplastic diseases.**
3. Changes in immune status. Age affects such changes, e.g., the loss of maternal immunity by the newborn, or the destruction of the immune system by immunosuppressive diseases, such as AIDS.
4. Changes in physiological reserve capacity and physiological resistance, i.e., aging. The very young and the very old, for example, are more susceptible to **enteric** and pneumonic infections, which are generally of little or no consequence to a healthy adolescent or adult.

Neoplastic diseases–relating to neoplasms or new growths of tissue that serve no physiological function, such as tumors.
Enteric–pertaining to the intestines.

Susceptibility–the degree to which a host lacks sufficient resistance to a particular pathogenic agent to prevent disease if or when exposed.

Resistance–the total of a host's mechanisms that pose barriers to the invasion or multiplication of infectious agents, or that prevent damage by an agent's toxic products.

Other host factors that are commonly considered include sex, ethnic group, social class, occupation, marital status, and birth order. These factors will be discussed in Chapter 7. Later in the text you will also come across the terms **susceptibility** and **resistance**. These are best considered as the two extremes on a biological continuum. They describe, for a population or for an individual, the current status vis-a-vis some disease process. They represent the final biological assessment of the host's condition after all host factors have been taken into consideration.

Biological Agent Factors Important to Preventive Medicine

Several biological characteristics of agents are important in understanding their importance to the study of epidemiology and their subsequent influence on the spread of disease throughout a community. For example, immunogenicity or the ability of an agent's antigens to provoke or initiate an immune response in an exposed host is a fundamental component in efforts to control disease. In regular measles (rubeola), the normal response of the body's immune system is to stimulate an appropriate antibody response to protect against subsequent attacks of the same disease while on the other hand, the agent that causes gonorrhea possesses little immunogenicity.

A general understanding of the environmental requirements and limitations of the agent or pathogenic organism against which preventive efforts are to be made is fundamental to the study of disease. It should be noted that temperature requirements, pH tolerance and predators and competitors are all important to understanding the pattern of disease and to identify essential focal points in attacking the chain of transmission.

Other key characteristics in understanding the dynamics of survival of microorganisms are host range, recrudescence/latency, and antigenic drift and shift.

With respect to extended host range, most infectious agents are not limited to one specific host species. To complicate public health control measures, as the number of host species in which the organism may find a safe refuge increase so do the problems associated with prevention, control and eradication. For example, St. Louis encephalitis involves many bird, mammalian, and mosquito species which hinders disease control. In contrast epidemic typhus involves one host (human) and one vector (body louse). Note also that rabies possesses a wide host range involving many species of animals (dogs, foxes, skunks, wolves, coyotes, opossums, cats, etc.).

Recrudescence and latency represent another phenomena that are associated with agents that represent another complicated problem for disease prevention control measures. For example, latency involves the ability of an agent to survive for extended periods of time within a host without producing clinical disease or whose presence is somewhat limited by being demonstrable by any of our current diagnostic procedures (i.e., herpes simplex, cold sores). While recrudescence, the reactivation of a latent or dormant infection to an active state, either inapparent (not noticeable) or associated with clinical disease also poses a problem for public health officials. Generally, the factors which precipitate recrudescence have not been well defined for most infections and have been nebulously termed as "stress."

Infections evidencing these properties include typhus, herpes simplex, and malaria to mention a few. One should note that this is an ideal mechanism for long term "silent" survival and widespread dissemination of disease.

Another unique survival mechanism of microorganisms involves antigenic drift and shift. Antigenic drift refers to a minor periodic and often annual alteration in the antigenic structure of the agent (microorganism) which may render prior immunity distinctively less effective. This event may be sufficient to minimally negate or significantly alter existing immunity within the host. However, when major alterations in the antigenic composition (major changes in the structure of the protein coat of the virus) occur, prior immunity may be rendered totally ineffective. This phenomena may be often observed in influenza epidemics when major changes in the antigenic composition of the virus occur resulting in serious outbreaks of influenza every nine to thirteen years. Epidemiologists generally are concerned with this phenomena as it impacts on public health programs designed to control influenza through vaccination programs.

Characteristics of Host-Agent Interaction

There are several important concepts involving the interactions between humans on other hosts, and their agents. These concepts (infectivity, pathogenicity, and virulence) will be discussed in this section.

Infectivity

Infectivity refers to the ability of an agent to establish infection once it is in contact with an individual member of the host species. Basically, the term implies the ability of an agent to lodge and multiply in the host. This concept is very important when epidemiologists are confronted with an outbreak of a disease and no overt or suspected agent has been identified (e.g., Legionnaire's disease when it was first discovered). Generally, infectivity varies with the age of the host, the portal of entry of the agent into the host, general host susceptibility, previous immunity, and so forth. For example, agents with high infectivity (assuming no prior immunity) include smallpox and regular measles, whereas agents that possess low infectivity include leprosy and histoplasmosis. Rabies is another disease in which the agent can readily establish an infection in a susceptible host.

Infectivity is measured by calculating a secondary attack rate as follows:

$$\text{Secondary attack rate (SAR)} = \frac{\begin{array}{c}\text{Number of persons developing}\\\text{disease within a reasonable}\\\text{incubation period following}\\\text{exposure minus the initial}\\\text{(primary) case}\end{array}}{\begin{array}{c}\text{Total number of persons}\\\text{exposed to the primary case}\\\text{during the same time period}\end{array}} \times 100$$

Pathogenicity

Pathogenicity is the ability of an agent to produce clinical disease once infection has been established. Generally, the expression of pathogenicity depends on how rapid the agent can multiply and whether or not the agent produces **toxins.** It should also be noted that, in many instances, no response by the host may result in no disease, for the agent may not, in and of itself, produce sufficient damage. Under laboratory conditions, pathogenicity can be measured as the proportion of individuals evidencing infection that sometimes become clinical cases. In actual field work, however, this is rarely possible. Agents possessing high pathogenicity include rabies, smallpox, AIDS, and regular measles. Agents with low pathogenicity include tuberculosis, poliomyelitis, and leprosy.

Toxins–any poisonous albumins or bases that are produced in the metabolisms of plant or animal organisms.

Virulence

Virulence denotes the ability of an agent to produce a severe clinical case of the disease and/or death. Epidemiologists use a measurement called the case fatality rate (CFR) to determine the proportion of individuals who are clinically ill from a certain disease and suffer the consequence of death during a reasonable time period. The CFR is determined as follows:

$$\text{CFR} = \frac{\text{Number of deaths during a specified period post onset}}{\text{Number of cases of clinical diseases diagnosed}} \times 100$$

The characteristics of host-agent interactions are important to epidemiologists in that they are essential in determining the patterns of disease occurrence as evaluated from a clinical perspective. For example, regular measles, rabies, smallpox, and other epidemic diseases of both humans and animals are all characterized by high infectivity, moderate to high pathogenicity, and a high degree of virulence. Second, because of these fundamental host-agent interactions, infections differ in their expression in a population, as can be seen in Figure 4.1.

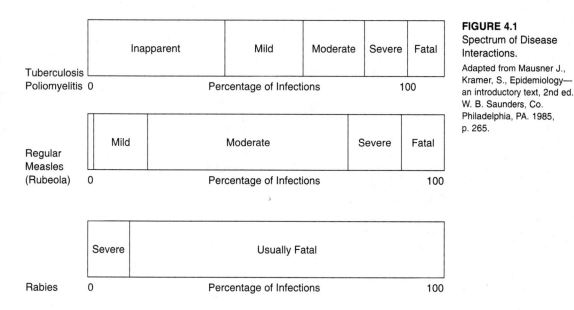

FIGURE 4.1
Spectrum of Disease Interactions.

Adapted from Mausner J., Kramer, S., Epidemiology— an introductory text, 2nd ed. W. B. Saunders, Co. Philadelphia, PA. 1985, p. 265.

Hosts as Carriers of Infection

As we learned in Chapter 3, the term *carrier* refers to an individual who is a "healthy shedder" of a microorganism and who serves as a source of infection for others. Carriers present a particularly difficult problem for control efforts, because clinically they appear "healthy" and, consequently, no steps are taken to treat their infection or to restrict their movement. There are four types of carriers.

Carriers with *inapparent infections* are individuals who have an infection but show no signs or symptoms. Such carriers occur with considerable frequency in many diseases. Epidemiological studies of poliomyelitis, for example, indicate that of one hundred individuals infected, one infected person will develop paralytic disease, four infected persons will develop nonparalytic disease, and ninety-five infections will remain inapparent. In the case of hepatitis A, the ratio of cases with jaundice to those not experiencing jaundice increases with age. As with poliomyelitis, the majority of cases of hepatitis A in young children result in inapparent infections, since jaundice is not a common manifestation in children. In children, there may be ten or more inapparent infections for each case of jaundice that develops. In adults, this ratio may be as high as 2 to 1 or 1 to 1. In the case of meningococcal meningitis, the carrier rate may be as high as 5 to 10 percent among community populations and considerably higher on military bases.

Incubatory carriers are those persons who are capable of transmitting an infection prior to the onset of signs and symptoms of the disease. For some diseases, incubatory carriers do not exist, while for other diseases such carriers may exist for months prior to the onset of illness. In hepatitis

B, the blood of infected persons may be infectious for as long as three months prior to the onset of jaundice. In dog rabies, the virus may be present in the saliva within five days prior to the onset of symptoms. The duration of the incubatory carrier state in rabies has been used to determine a satisfactory holding time, of seven to ten days, for dogs that have bitten humans. If a dog does not develop the signs and symptoms of rabies within this time, there is little likelihood that infection was transmitted as a result of the bite.

Convalescent carriers are those individuals who, after experiencing acute illness, continue to be infectious during and after their return to health. In many diseases, a small percentage of individuals will be found to be infectious during and after the convalescent period. For example, the improper use of drugs in treating salmonellosis patients has been found to increase the likelihood of a patient becoming a convalescent carrier.

Chronic carriers are those individuals who continue to harbor infectious agents for a year or more. This situation is encountered in typhoid fever, viral hepatitis, shigellosis, and other diseases. The percentage of infected individuals who become chronic carriers is quite small (Centers for Disease Control 1987).

Summary

This chapter explores the role of host factors and their influence on human health and disease. Host factors are analyzed by determining if an association between the presence of a factor and the occurrence of a disease are statistically significant. Association between a factor and the occurrence of an illness is often described by calculating an attack rate.

An understanding of the biological characteristics of agents is important in regard to prevention efforts. Such characteristics aid in establishing specific points to interrupt the chain of transmission of disease.

Infectivity, pathogenicity and virulence are major concepts in determining how infection may express itself in population groups and aid epidemiologists as they try to fully understand the dynamics of disease and injury in our society.

Discussion Questions

1. Describe how age is related to disease. What factors are of primary importance in attempting to relate age to the expression of disease?
2. Describe the major biological agent factors important to preventive medicine.
3. Define the following terms: infectivity, pathogenicity, and virulence. How are they measured?

4. Describe the different types of carriers and how they pose problems with respect to the control of disease.
5. Define and explain an attack rate.

References

Centers for Disease Control. 1987. Training publication 3030-G. Atlanta, GA: U.S. Department of Health and Human Services.

Duncan, D. 1988. *Epidemiology: Basis for disease prevention and health promotion.* New York: Macmillan.

Friedman, G. 1974. *Primer of epidemiology.* New York: McGraw-Hill.

Mausner, J., and S. Kramer. 1985. *Epidemiology: An introductory text.* Philadelphia: W. B. Saunders.

Roht, L., B. Selwyn, A. Holguin, and B. Christensen. 1982. *Principles of epidemiology: A self-testing guide.* New York: Academic Press.

CHAPTER 5

Environmental Factors in Health and Illness

Introduction

Environment–the surroundings of a living organism. For human beings the environment is comprised of physical, biological, and cultural components.

In terms of human health, the **environment** is the surroundings of a human being. Humans have a need to establish an equilibrium, or homeostasis, with their environment. Indeed, life depends on the continuous interaction between a human and his or her environment. To travel into space, astronauts must take with them the essentials of the environment on earth—air to breathe, water and food, clothing to maintain body temperature, and so on. Our environment makes life possible and also helps to determine the quality of our lives. Some knowledge of the complexity of the environment is essential to epidemiologists. They need to understand: (1) why continued human life and health depend on the conservation of environmental qualities; (2) how the environment directly and indirectly causes and conditions health and illness; and (3) why epidemiology faces a formidable task in the search for and prevention of the environmental causes of illness. We will begin by discussing the physical, biological, and cultural components of the environment.

Components of the Environment

The Physical Environment

This component includes the physical and chemical surroundings of air, land, and sea. It also includes physical constants, such as gravity; geographical variables, such as soils, climate, altitude, and continentality; and energy from the sun and from stocks of fossil materials, such as coal and oil. The physical environment provides the sunlight, water, and air essential for life as well as the variety of land and seascapes that delight the eye and provide places for work and leisure. The physical environment also includes risks to health, such as overexposure to sunlight, severe climates, falling from high places, a shortage of clean air or water, earthquakes, floods, and volcanic eruptions.

The Biological Environment

This comprises all living things—plants, animals, and microbes living in or on the soil, in the air, and in water. Living things form communities in places in the physical environment. There is a distinct geographical distribution of these communities, according to land, water, altitude, and climate. Thus, the plant and animal communities of the humid tropics are quite different from those of the arctic.

The biological environment provides human populations with many of the conditions that make life possible. Plants convert solar energy to sugar energy through photosynthesis, which provides food energy for human and animal life and helps maintain the oxygen content of the atmosphere. Plants also supply wood for shelter and fuel, chemicals, oils, dyes, drugs, perfumes, paper, and many other materials for human technology. Animals provide meat, milk, hides, fur, casein, and other chemical compounds; they also serve as transport and motive power for human activities. Microbes are important in human digestion and in preparing and conserving food, such as in yeasts for breads and bacterial cultures for cheeses. The biological environment also contains agents of illness. The most formidable agents are the pathogenic viruses, bacteria, protozoa, and helminths that cause infectious diseases, and the insect vectors that transmit them; plant and animal poisons are other biological agents.

The Cultural Environment

This is the environment created by human culture—the social settings, the institutions and organizations of societies, and the transformations humans have made to the physical and biological environment, as in cities, farmlands, parks, and artificial lakes. Culture includes knowledge about when and how to behave in a social context, how to use tools, how to capture energy and food, and how to transmit knowledge to others. There are many different human cultures and there are many subcultures within every culture. All cultures have the knowledge accumulated over generations, which guides the perceptions and behaviors of individuals and groups in ways that generally support the societies in their environment. Cultural environments that provide congenial social situations, protection from hazards, clean living conditions, meaningful work, leisure time, education, and health and medical services are protective of public health. On the other hand, cultural environments can also promote illness and death, through social injustice or unrest, violence and war, poverty and ignorance, and hazardous worksites.

Other Concepts of Environment

Environment as Ecosystem

The physical, biological, and cultural components of the environment, including all living things, exist as a single life-supporting system, or

Ecosystem–an evolving system of populations of living things, their behavior, and environment, organized and functioning at levels of interaction that support life.

ecosystem. All things in the system are interdependent in some way, and changes in one will affect the others. This is why the environmental factors associated with health and illness are difficult to isolate for study and are unlikely to be the sole determinant in a cause-or-effect relationship. The agents that are necessary to cause an illness are always conditioned by other environmental factors and situations; by themselves, environmental agents are not usually sufficient to cause illness. Also necessary for illness is a susceptible host, a suitable environment for transmission, and the coincidence of all necessary and conditional factors in time and place. When epidemiologists study environmental factors that appear to be associated with health and illness, they analyze the factors as components of ecosystems, so that the interrelationships between factors are accounted for (Green 1990).

Environment as Place

Plants and animals live as communities in particular geographical locations. Major plant associations (biomes), such as tropical rainforests, grasslands, and subarctic taiga, form habitats for particular associations of animals, which are then more or less confined to these locations. Human populations, through their cultural development of such things as food supplies and storage, artificial heating and cooling, and transportation, are not confined to particular habitats but have come to settle in all varieties of the earth's environment from the arctic to the tropics and from the seashore to high mountains. Most people, however, are not nomads or travelers and tend to spend all or most of their lives in or near the **place** where they were born. The places where human communities live have, over many generations, come to acquire a distinctive physical, biological, and cultural character to their environment, with the cultural characteristics often being the most evident. As a traveler crosses the border between Texas and Mexico, or flies from India to Switzerland, there are marked differences between the places, in the way the respective human cultures have organized and used the landscapes; created economies, religions, and other institutions; and developed their own life-styles. These different places are the contexts for human health and illness.

Place–a geographical location on the earth's surface that has cultural meaning to human populations; it is usually inhabited by a community and has a settlement name.

Self-Specific Environments

The environment shared by a group of people is called a place in geographical terms, but each person has a *self-specific environment*. In theory, a person lives in an environment that is unique in terms of where and how one's time is spent and the kinds of interactions that go on between a person and their surroundings. People may share the same time and place, but the use of the time and the place varies from person to person. Most adults spend, on the average, 8 hours of their 24-hour day sleeping; 8 hours working; 6 hours doing things at home; 1½ hours shopping, visiting, and in other things away from home; and ½ hour traveling. But a farmer and a schoolteacher in the same place have different environments for work; a farmer in Zimbabwe in Africa has a different environment from one in Canada. Self-specific environments take on special meaning when we are concerned with groups of people who have been exposed to particular environments that may be hazardous to their health, such as shipyard workers who have been exposed to asbestos and the risk of cancer.

Another dimension to environmental patterns is that they change over time. The situation in a particular place in 1995 may be different from what it was in 1965 with respect to factors related to health and illness. Populations also change with time, but each generation tends to retain many of the characteristics of its youth, such as the immunities to diseases experienced as children and dietary preferences. Thus, the group of people born in the 1960s (a **cohort**) tends to have many things in common, such as dietary preferences, which differ from those of earlier or later cohorts all living in the same place.

The Bodily Environment

The human body has an internal environment of passages that forms an intimate contact with the surrounding environment. The most important of these passages are the respiratory tract, in contact with air, and the digestive tract, in contact with food and drink. The skin and the senses of sight, sound, touch, and smell are also important for communication with the physical, biological, and social nature of our surroundings. Through these pathways move most of the factors that cause physical and mental illness. The only exceptions are genetic factors, which are determined at conception.

The First Environment

The first environment that all of us experience is the womb. Although this is an unconscious experience, it is one of the most important in conditioning health and other capacities throughout life. The environment of the unborn infant includes the nutrients transferred from the mother's bloodstream, antibodies to resist infectious agents, and perhaps ingredients from tobacco, alcohol, and other chemicals that the mother may consume. The environment outside the mother may directly affect the fetus, as with exposure to ionizing radiations or to excessive vibration.

The environment shortly after birth begins to include the conscious perception of one's surroundings and the beginning of the process of socialization. For example, while breastfeeding provides nutrients, it also lays the foundation for psychological and social development. Infants who are deprived of normal motherly caring in the first months of life are more likely to have social and behavioral difficulties later in life. This early environment is crucial in establishing the appropriate conditions under which optimal growth and development will occur.

As the infant becomes a child, the power of perception is increased. The environment is seen, felt, heard, and smelled. There is color, shape,

Cohort–originally referred to a group of persons born the same year in the same place. Today, the term is used for any group that is followed up over time. Research subjects are selected for inclusion in a cohort because of some current exposure to a possible cause of illness, and they are subsequently followed up over time to measure the incidence of the disease being investigated. Cohort studies are also known as incidence studies or prospective studies.

size, texture, time, and space. There are feelings for surroundings, such as cool or warm, soothing or sinister, safe or dangerous. At the same time, our parents and others teach us how to interpret these perceptions according to our culture. Children acquire language skills and education in the social arrangements, institutions, and technologies of their society. But they do not all obtain this information in the same way. Children born into affluent, well-educated homes, for example, have different opportunities for education and health than children born into poorer, less-endowed homes.

The social and economic differences in human populations now account for a large portion of the differences between countries in terms of health and illness. In well-developed Western countries, where data on occupational social class is collected, there is a definite gradient in mortality rates between upper- and lower-class levels, with the highest mortality rates being in the category of unskilled manual workers (Table 5.1). Many environmental factors are involved in this difference besides occupation and income; these include education, diet, exercise, quality of housing, and access to services such as medical care.

Similar contrasts between those more and less affluent are found in the less industrialized countries of South America, Africa, and Asia. In these countries, the proportion of the population that is in the least skilled occupational groups—with low income, little or no formal education, and

TABLE 5.1 Mortality and Social Class in the United Kingdom, 1980, and in New Zealand, 1982

		United Kingdom		New Zealand
		Men[1]	Married Women[1]	Both Sexes[1]
Social Class		SMR[2]	SMR[2]	SMR[2]
I	Higher professional, managerial	77	82	90
II	Lower professional, managerial	81	87	99
IIIa	Other nonmanual	99	92	99
IIIb	Skilled manual	106	115	
IV	Semiskilled manual	114	119	104
V	Unskilled manual	137	135	107

Source: Data on United Kingdom from: Great Britain Working Group on Inequalities in Health. 1980. *Inequalities in health: Report of a research working group*. London: Department of Health and Social Security. Data on New Zealand from: Hyslop, J., J. Dowland, and J. Hickling. 1983. *Health facts: New Zealand*. Wellington, New Zealand: Department of Health.

[1] 15–64 year age group.
[2] SMR is the standardized mortality ratio, an age-adjusted percentage rate of mortality where 100 is the national average. Thus, in the table, an SMR of 77 means that the ratio is 23 percent lower than the national average, and an SMR of 137 is 37 percent higher (see Chapter 7 for a definition of the SMR).

Environmental Factors in Health and Illness

least access to social and medical services—is much greater. They often live in poorer housing without piped clean water, sewerage systems, garbage collection services, electricity for refrigeration, and other amenities that help protect against infectious diseases. In these environments, malnutrition, diarrheal diseases, typhoid fever, cholera, and parasitic infections are likely to be prevalent. Especially susceptible to malnutrition and infections are infants and children. While significant improvements were made between 1950 and 1990 in reducing death from infectious diseases in poorer communities in all countries, a very large proportion of deaths in the world is still among children under the age of five years. The percentage of deaths in this age group ranges from less than 1 percent in Sweden to over 80 percent in Malawi (Table 5.2).

Epidemiology and Geography

As discussed in Chapter 3, the environment is an important consideration in any epidemiological study. It conditions the state of health of individuals and of populations and is the context of the agents that cause illness. Although human behaviors are becoming increasingly important in the **etiology** and prevention of many illnesses, the environment will continue to be the origin of infectious diseases and the context of illnesses of all kinds (Moeller 1992).

Etiology–the science of the causes or origins of disease.

TABLE 5.2 Percentage of Total Deaths Occurring in Children under Five Years of Age, Selected Countries, by Region

Region	Country	Year	Percentage
Africa	Egypt	1981	38.4
	Malawi	1977	80.4
	Zimbabwe	1982	32.4
N. America	Canada	1987	1.8
	Cuba	1986	4.4
	Mexico	1985	21.4
	United States	1986	2.2
S. America	Brazil	1986	18.8
	Colombia	1986	14.9
Asia	Bangladesh	1982	48.0
	Japan	1987	1.2
	Jordan	1980	26.4
	Pakistan	1985	54.1
	Thailand	1987	6.9
Europe	France	1987	1.4
	Italy	1984	1.5
	Poland	1987	3.2
	Sweden	1987	0.8
Oceania	Australia	1986	2.3
	New Zealand	1987	2.4

Source: Data from United Nations. 1990. *Demographic yearbook 1988.* New York: U.N.

The geographical distribution of disease has, for centuries, been an indicator of the importance of the environment in conditioning health in populations. The ancient Greeks, for example, observed that some places had higher frequencies of illnesses than others, and that some places had climates and food supplies that seemed to offer healthier living than others. Modern maps of the distribution of infectious diseases are largely a reflection of the cultural capacities to control those diseases. The map of malaria in 1990 (Figure 5.1) shows this disease to be largely confined to the tropics. A map for 1940, though, would show malaria to be prevalent in parts of the southern United States and southwestern Europe as well; and a map for 1840 would show that malaria was endemic in the Mississippi and Ohio river valleys, the southern part of the United States, and most of Europe. These geographical changes are largely a result of human modifications to the environment of the mosquito vector for malaria. These modifications were comparatively inexpensive and long-lasting in the subtropics but have proven much more difficult to achieve in the tropics. There are more species of mosquito vectors in the tropics and they thrive in much greater numbers; mean temperatures are higher throughout the year and favor transmission year round; and the human populations are primarily rural and more dispersed.

The geographical distribution of some noninfectious diseases suggests that the environment, or differences in the behavior or biology of populations in geographical environments, also has a major role in their etiology. The incidence of major cancers, for example, varies strikingly from one part of the world to another. In 1987, cancers of the lung in males occurred with the highest frequency in the United States, with a rate of 110 per 100,000, and with the lowest frequency in India, with a rate of 5.8, a nineteen-fold difference. Other rates for comparison are given in Table 5.3. When we look at the incidence rates for cancers of the lung in males and females by country, we see a marked geographical variation worldwide (Figure 5.2). In the case of lung cancer, we know that the variation is, in large part, explained by the history of the use of cigarettes. Other cancer sites display their own distinctive geographical patterns. The magnitude of these differences in rates indicates that environmental and behavioral factors are foremost in causing major cancers, rather than genetic or other biological characteristics of populations.

Environmental Risk Factors and Agents

As defined in Chapter 3, a risk factor is an environmental or behavioral factor that is associated with increasing the risk of a particular illness or of death. The degree to which a risk factor causes illness or death has not usually been established, although there are ways of estimating it (see Chapter 8). An agent is a known causal factor, as was discussed in Chapter 3. The environment is the context of all risk factors and agents, known and unknown.

Environmental Factors in Health and Illness

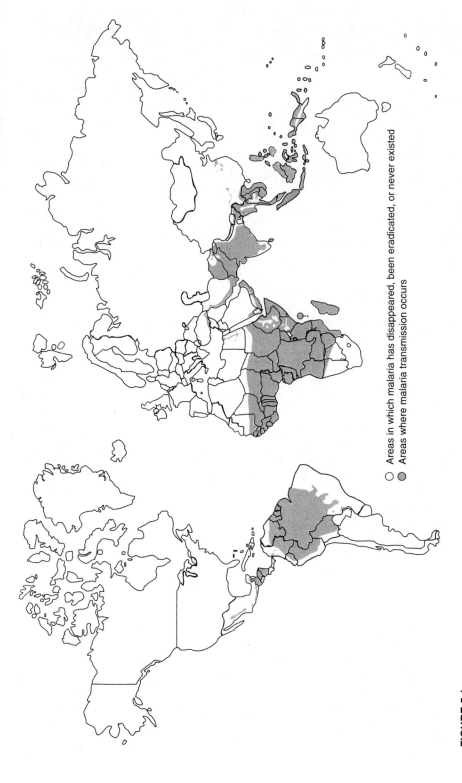

FIGURE 5.1
World Distribution of
Malaria, 1990.

Source: Used with
permission of the World
Health Organization.

○ Areas in which malaria has disappeared, been eradicated, or never existed
● Areas where malaria transmission occurs

TABLE 5.3 Comparison of Highest and Lowest Recorded Rates of Cancer Incidence from 96 World Registries for the Ten Most Frequent Sites in Males and in Females

	Males				Females		
Site	*High*	*Low*	*Ratio*	*Site*	*High*	*Low*	*Ratio*
Lung	110.0	5.8	19x	Breast	93.9	14.0	7x
Prostate	91.2	1.3	70x	Cervix	83.2	3.0	28x
Stomach	82.0	4.1	20x	Lung	68.1	0.5	136x
Oesophagus	35.8	0.6	60x	Stomach	36.6	1.6	23x
Liver	34.4	0.1	344x	Colon	29.0	0.7	41x
Colon	34.1	0.2	170x	Corpus uteri	25.2	1.2	21x
Nasopharynx	30.0	0.2	150x	Gallbladder	23.6	0.2	118x
Bladder	27.8	1.7	16x	Thyroid	18.2	0.1	182x
Rectum	22.6	1.5	15x	Rectum	15.9	1.3	12x
Pancreas	16.4	0.7	23x	Mouth	15.7	0.1	157x
All sites*	400.1	71.9	5x	All sites*	353.7	72.0	5x

Source: Data from Muir, C., J. Waterhouse, T. Mack, J. Powell, and S. Whelan. 1987. *Cancer incidence in five continents*, Vol. V. IARC Sci. Pub. No. 88. Lyon, France: International Agency for Research on Cancer.

Note: Rates are per 100,000 population age-adjusted to the World Standard Population. The reporting period ranges from 1977 to 1982, but most registries reported for 1978–1982. Rates based on less than ten cases are excluded.

*Skin cancers other than melanoma are excluded.

In practice, epidemiologists deal with specific problems and specific interrelations with the environment. They cannot deal with the complexities of entire ecosystems. They focus on specific problems, usually in the context of local communities or regional populations and within the time frames of a few months or years. In recent years, however, epidemiologists have become more involved with other scientists in assessing the risks associated with global pollution. For example, the increase in the amounts of carbon dioxide in the atmosphere, which may raise global temperatures, and the increase in the penetration of ultraviolet rays through the ozone layer in the stratosphere, which has been damaged by the human release of fluorocarbons, both pose long-term threats to human health. In the following sections, we will discuss some specific examples of environmental risk factors and agents that can lead to specific illnesses.

Biological

These include the agents of infectious disease (viruses, bacteria, protozoa, etc.), as described in Chapter 3, and the arthropod vectors that transmit some of them, such as mosquitoes for malaria, filariasis, and hemorrhagic fever; flies for river blindness (onchocerciasis), African trypanosomiasis, and shigellosis; ticks for Lyme disease and Rocky Mountain spotted fever; and fleas for plague and typhus. Also included are the animal hosts and reservoirs for the zoonotic infectious diseases, which are transmittable from vertebrate animals to humans.

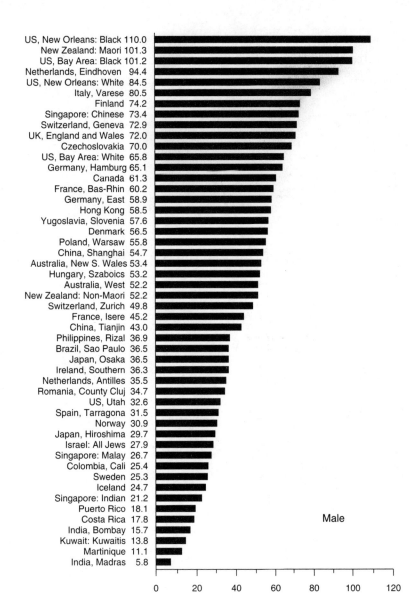

FIGURE 5.2

A, Incidence of Lung Cancer in 50 Populations.

Source: Data from Muir, C., J. Waterhouse, T. Mack, J. Powell, and S. Whelan. 1987. *Cancer incidence in five continents, Vol. V.* IARC Sci. Pub. No. 88. Lyon, France: International Agency for Research on Cancer.

Infectious disease agents continue to be discovered. In the last twenty years several previously unknown biological agents have been identified, including the viruses that cause AIDS, Ebola-Marburg disease, and Lassa fever, and the bacteria that causes legionellosis.

Food and Diet

The food patterns and dietary habits of populations are a reflection of many factors: their dependence on local environments to support a

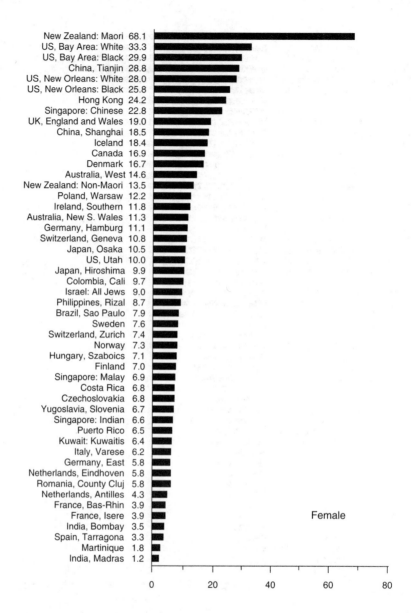

FIGURE 5.2

B, Incidence of Lung Cancer in 50 Populations.

Source: Data from Muir, C., J. Waterhouse, T. Mack, J. Powell, and S. Whelan. 1987. *Cancer incidence in five continents, Vol. V.* IARC Sci. Pub. No. 88. Lyon, France: International Agency for Research on Cancer.

New Zealand: Maori	68.1
US, Bay Area: White	33.3
US, Bay Area: Black	29.9
China, Tianjin	28.8
US, New Orleans: White	28.0
US, New Orleans: Black	25.8
Hong Kong	24.2
Singapore: Chinese	22.8
UK, England and Wales	19.0
China, Shanghai	18.5
Iceland	18.4
Canada	16.9
Denmark	16.7
Australia, West	14.6
New Zealand: Non-Maori	13.5
Poland, Warsaw	12.2
Ireland, Southern	11.8
Australia, New S. Wales	11.3
Germany, Hamburg	11.1
Switzerland, Geneva	10.8
Japan, Osaka	10.5
US, Utah	10.0
Japan, Hiroshima	9.9
Colombia, Cali	9.7
Israel: All Jews	9.0
Philippines, Rizal	8.7
Brazil, Sao Paulo	7.9
Sweden	7.6
Switzerland, Zurich	7.4
Norway	7.3
Hungary, Szaboics	7.1
Finland	7.0
Singapore: Malay	6.9
Costa Rica	6.8
Czechoslovakia	6.8
Yugoslavia, Slovenia	6.7
Singapore: Indian	6.6
Puerto Rico	6.5
Kuwait: Kuwaitis	6.4
Italy, Varese	6.2
Germany, East	5.8
Netherlands, Eindhoven	5.8
Romania, County Cluj	5.8
Netherlands, Antilles	4.3
France, Bas-Rhin	3.9
France, Isere	3.9
India, Bombay	3.5
Spain, Tarragona	3.3
Martinique	1.8
India, Madras	1.2

Female

particular pattern of agriculture; their economic capacity to import a variety of foodstuffs from other places; their local cultural preferences for food and customs in eating; and individual behavioral patterns and choices of diet. It is a combination of environment and social and individual behavior that conditions diet.

Epidemiologists have identified several dietary risk factors, including saturated fats and cholesterol for heart disease; childhood consumption of salted marine fish for cancer of the nasopharynx (a disease of major importance in some Chinese populations); excessive caloric and high fat diets for obesity; and alcoholic drinks for diseases of the liver and cancers of the upper digestive tract. Agents that cause nutritional deficiency disease by their *absence* include iron for iron deficiency anemia, niacin for pellagra, calcium for bone and tooth deformities, and vitamin D for rickets. Certain dietary factors have been associated with having a protective effect for some diseases, that is, with a reduction in disease risk. Fresh fruits rich in vitamin C, and fresh green cruciferous and yellow/red vegetables rich in carotene, have been associated with a reduced risk of cancers of the stomach and colon.

Pollution

Air, water, and food that become polluted with chemical or biological waste from industrial, agricultural, transportational, or domestic activities can contain environmental agents and risk factors. Urban air often contains moderate amounts of carbon monoxide, which comes from automobile and industrial exhausts and is a risk factor for newborn infants and for individuals with heart disease (Watson, Bates, and Kennedy 1988). Water supplies can become contaminated with disease-causing organisms from human or animal fecal waste, with nitrates in agricultural areas where nitrogen fertilizer is used, and with a variety of chemicals from industrial and domestic waste dumps that have entered ground or surface waters. Such contaminations lead to infectious diarrheal disease and a variety of chronic noninfectious diseases and allergies. Foods contaminated by pesticides, lead from auto and industrial exhausts, and biological organisms such as salmonella also cause a variety of illnesses.

Radiation

For populations with fair skins, outdoor occupations, a preference for sunbathing, and exposure to intense sunlight are risk factors for skin cancer. Overexposure to artificial tanning lamps poses a similar risk. Ionizing radiations from uncontrolled sources, such as the accidental discharge of radioactive steam at a nuclear power station, or radioactive fallout from the atmospheric explosions of nuclear weapons, are agents of radiation injuries and cancers. High dosages of and direct exposure to radiation tend to produce immediate injurious effects, while lower dosages and indirect exposures lead to cancers that may take years to develop (Beebe 1982).

Natural Hazards

As populations increase in size and density around the world, the hazards posed by earthquakes, floods, tsunamis, hurricanes, tornadoes, and volcanic activity have tended to increase (Bernstein, Baxter, and Buist 1986). The epidemiology of these hazards is an expanding field of knowledge. Although this field of study may contribute little toward understanding the causes of these events, it is helping us to understand how human behaviors, settlement forms, and other environmental modifications can affect the risk of injury and death, and how to evaluate the effectiveness of emergency services.

Occupational

The environment of work is of particular importance because it can expose individuals to many agents and risk factors (Monson 1990). Some occupational agents cause immediate illness, such as an on-the-job injury, and have varying times for rehabilitation. Other work injuries cause permanent disabilities, such as the loss of hearing, sight, and limb, or paralysis from a spinal injury. Some diseases appear decades later, often long after the person affected has left the job responsible for the disease. This is the case with most job-related cancers.

Certain occupations have clearly established health risks, such as the associations of silicosis and tuberculosis with mining, byssinosis with cotton dust in textile industries, and severe injuries with the construction industry, deep-sea fishing, and ocean oil mining. These illnesses occur in comparatively large groups of workers, and they occur often enough to clearly associate them with the occupation. In interpreting occupational risk, however, epidemiologists need to control for various factors, such as educational level, socioeconomic status, gender differences, and other risk behaviors, as these may play a confounding role.

Occupational cancers have been more difficult to identify and associate with particular occupations, because of the long latent periods between the time of exposure to causal agents and the time of diagnosis. By linking records of cancer incidence with records of occupation, and by compiling detailed job histories, epidemiologists have identified several rare cancers as being of very high risk for specific occupations. These include exposure to asbestos with mesothelioma, exposure to wood dust in the joinery trade with cancer of the nasal sinuses, exposure to benzene in a variety of trades with cancer of the bladder, and exposure to polyvinyl chloride gas in the manufacture of certain plastics with cancer of the liver. Occupational environments that are excessively hot or cold, that have loud or monotonous noise, or require working in the same posture or with the same muscles for hours at a time may also lead to a variety of physical and psychological ailments.

Recreational

Modern societies engage in very high risk activities, such as hang gliding, diving, hunting, motorcycle and car racing, snowmobiling, and contact sports. American football, basketball, ice hockey, and baseball contribute to a substantial number of injuries and some deaths each year. Together with individual behavior, the environment of these activities is a major component in the risks involved. Epidemiology helps to identify specific risks, and, where possible, the environment of these activities can then be modified to reduce certain risks, such as removing specific hazards where recreations are carried out, improving the safety of equipment, and regulating how, when and where the activities are conducted.

Social

Different social groups and societies create social environments that influence individuals to behave in ways that affect their health, or that impose psychological stress or physical violence. For the most part, social environments are important positive influences on health as, for example, in the normal family support of children, or in social support of the elderly and disabled. Some social environments, though, are agents and risk factors for illnesses, such as the social customs of drinking alcohol, smoking tobacco, sniffing glue, and snorting cocaine. All addictions are socially encouraged by peer pressures of various kinds; biological differences between individuals make some people more susceptible to addiction than others. Some social situations involving power and injustice lead to the oppression of individuals, which in turn can lead to mental illness. Other situations promote violence, as in the form of child and spouse battering, assault, suicide, rape, and homicide. Handguns in American society have become a major risk factor for homicide, which is now a leading cause of death in the 15–35-year age group (see Chapter 7). Also, violent incidents such as the 1995 bombing of the Oklahoma City Federal Building may reflect or be prompted by anger and distrust of our social and political institutions.

Summary

The environment—the physical, biological, and cultural surroundings of human beings—is essential in supporting life. It conditions the quality of living and the status of health for populations. The conservation of those environmental qualities that have become essential to life through evolution is vital for human survival. The environment is the context of all the agents and risk factors that cause or increase illness and death. Specific agents and risk factors have been identified in a wide range of environmental settings, including biological, food and diet, pollution, radiation, natural hazards, occupational, recreational, and social.

Discussion Questions

1. What are some of the qualities of the environment that are essential to human life and health?
2. In your own surroundings, identify physical, biological, and cultural components. What are some of the ways in which they are interacting?

3. Review the kinds of agents that cause illness, which were discussed in Chapter 3. How does the environment condition the ways these agents may interact with populations of human beings to cause illness?
4. Think of the occupations and recreations that are common in your own community. What illnesses are most likely to occur in these occupations? Try to obtain information from your library to confirm your findings.

References

Beebe, G. W. Ionizing radiation and health. 1982. *American Scientist* 70:35–44.

Bernstein, R. S., P. J. Baxter, and A. S. Buist. 1986. Introduction to the epidemiological aspects of explosive volcanism. *American Journal of Public Health.* 76:3–9, supplement.

Green, L. W. 1990. *Community health,* 6th ed. St. Louis: Times/Mirror Mosby.

Moeller, D. W. 1992. *Environmental health.* Cambridge: Harvard University Press.

Monson, R. R. 1990. *Occupational epidemiology,* 2nd ed. Boca Raton, FL: CRC Press.

Watson, A. Y., R. R. Bates, and D. Kennedy, eds. 1988. *Air pollution, the automobile, and public health.* Washington, D.C.: National Academy Press.

CHAPTER 6

The Measurement of Illness and Death

Introduction

Measuring the occurrence of illness (morbidity) and death (mortality) is of primary importance in epidemiology. Epidemiologists must analyze such data in order to investigate the causes of illness and death and to devise preventive measures. Illness is used here as it was defined in Chapter 3, that is, to include all known causes of ill-health—disease, injuries, addictions, nutritional disorders, congenital anomalies, allergies, and mental illnesses. Many of these same causes of illness may lead to death and be referred to as causes of death. The causes of illness and death are classified by an international statistical classification, under the direction of the World Health Organization (Table 3.1).

Data on the occurrence of various illnesses in populations are rarely complete. It is neither practical nor necessary to collect information on the occurrence of every known illness episode, from the common cold to cancer of the lung, or from a minor cut to a severe injury. Special studies have been conducted from time to time in selected communities to measure the full extent of illness, and these are sufficient to describe general patterns. Some populations have been studied more closely than others, for example, schoolchildren, workers in selected industries, and residents of institutions such as hospitals and prisons. Some countries have conducted comprehensive illness surveys, which collect much detailed information at one time but at considerable cost, such as the Canada Health Survey of 1978–79. Other countries opt for the regular collection of limited information, such as the U.S. National Health Survey, which takes a small sample of the population in each state to collect data on the frequency of acute and chronic conditions, lost work and school time due to illness, and physician and hospital visits.

The occurrence of certain infectious and noninfectious diseases is well-documented, because physicians and other health professionals are required to report every case that is diagnosed. Eight infectious diseases are universally notifiable to the World Health Organization: plague, cholera, yellow fever, louseborne typhus fever, relapsing fever, paralytic poliomyelitis, malaria, and viral influenza (Benenson 1990). Other kinds of infectious disease cases are reported only to national or state health authorities.

Certain noninfectious diseases, such as cancer, have special registries to record all known cases in defined populations. In the United States there are thirty-five registries in certain states and major cities. Only a few small nations have national registries, including Finland, Iceland, New Zealand, Norway, and Singapore. Information on nonfatal injuries and other causes of illness comes mostly from hospitals and mental health centers. Police and ambulance records provide data on injuries from motor-vehicle crashes; fire departments provide data on fire-related injuries. There are also some surveillance systems that provide limited data on injuries related to occupations, sports, and consumer products.

The occurrence of death is comparatively well-reported and documented. All countries have systems for collecting vital statistics that include the factual occurrence of a birth or a death. In most well-developed countries, almost 100 percent of all deaths have the cause of death reported; however, in some cases, the cause of death may be erroneously reported. In most less-developed countries, where the accurate determination of death is largely confined to major cities with hospitals, the cause of death may be reported only 10 to 40 percent of the time. The accuracy of determination depends on the cause of death—the cause in a car crash is simpler to determine than the cause of a fever of unknown origin—on the experience and skill of the person making the determination, and on the availability and completeness of the medical history of the dead person. For difficult cases, an autopsy generally yields the most reliable information on cause of death, but only a small proportion of deaths are autopsied in all countries (Gobbato et al. 1982). In the United States about 12 percent of all deaths have an autopsy, a proportion that has been slowly declining in recent years.

The causes of death are recorded on a death certificate, which follows a standard format. The immediate cause of death is recorded first, and then the conditions, if any, that gave rise to the immediate cause. Two such conditions may be reported, and these are referred to as the secondary cause and underlying cause, respectively. The underlying cause is most often recorded in official statistics as the cause of death (Gittelsohn 1982). In recent years, it has been recognized that this practice of reporting leads to a bias in accounting for the impact of some conditions that cause death. Diabetes mellitus, for example, is more often reported as a secondary cause than as an underlying cause and thus appears in statistical tables as being of lesser importance. The solution to this is to compile data on all the causes reported on death certificates, a practice that has been followed in the United States since 1975.

Key Sources and Types of Data

The World Health Organization has listed the following as key sources of surveillance data (World Health Organization 1988):

1. Mortality reports
2. Morbidity reports
3. Epidemic reports
4. Reports of laboratory utilization (including laboratory test results)
5. Reports of individual case investigations
6. Reports of epidemic investigations
7. Special surveys (e.g., hospital admissions, disease registers, and serologic surveys)
8. Information on animal reservoirs and vectors
9. Demographic data
10. Environmental data

Some of these sources of data are collected as part of a surveillance system. Others are collected for different reasons but may be used for surveillance purposes. The most common sources of data are described in the following sections.

Mortality Data

Vital Statistics.   Vital statistics include data on birth, death, marriage, and divorce. Such records may be available at the local and state level within a matter of days or weeks, but they are not always coded or computerized. The Centers for Disease Control and Prevention's National Center for Health Statistics (NCHS) collects a monthly national sample of death certificates and publishes a report based on these sample data three months later. The NCHS also provides complete national mortality data within two to three years. Approximately 121 cities around the United States report to CDCP the number of deaths by age from all causes combined, and from pneumonia or influenza, within about three weeks of occurrence. These data are published the following week in the Morbidity and Mortality Weekly Report (MMWR).

Medical Examiner Data.   Coroners and medical examiners can provide information on sudden or unexpected deaths. Their reports are available at the state or county level; these reports often include details about the cause and nature of death that are not found on the death certificate.

Morbidity Data

Notifiable Disease Reports.   Each state government establishes by law what health events must be reported by health care providers in that state. Some states require that as few as 35 conditions be reported; others require as many as 130 conditions. Most states also require that an outbreak of any condition be reported. Table 6.1 lists the conditions that are reportable in many states. As that table shows, reportable conditions are

TABLE 6.1 Infectious Diseases Designated as Notifiable at the National Level—United States, 1994

AIDS	Hepatitis, unspecified	Rocky Mountain
Amebiasis*	Legionellosis	spotted fever (Typhus
Anthrax	Leprosy (Hansen's disease)	fever, tickborne)
Aseptic meningitis	Leptospirosis	Rubella
Botulism	Lyme disease	Salmonellosis*
Brucellosis	Lymphogranuloma	Shigellosis*
Chancroid*	venereum*	Syphilis
Cholera	Malaria	Syphilis, congenital
Congenital rubella syndrome	Measles	Tetanus
Diphtheria	Meningococcal infection	Toxic shock syndrome
Encephalitis	Mumps	Trichinosis
Escherichia coli O157:H7*	Pertussis	Tuberculosis
Gonorrhea	Plague	Tularemia
Granuloma inguinale*	Poliomyelitis	Typhoid fever
Haemophilus influenza	Psittacosis	Varicella (chicken
Hepatitis A	Rabies, animal	pox)*†
Hepatitis B	Rabies, human	Yellow fever*
Hepatitis, non-A, non-B	Rheumatic fever*	

Source: Centers for Disease Control. Atlanta, GA. *Morbidity and Mortality Weekly Report* 43:43, 1994.
*Reports of these diseases are not printed weekly in Table I or Table II of the *MMWR*.
†Although varicella is not officially a nationally notifiable disease, the Council of State and Territorial Epidemiologists encourages transmission of information about cases of varicella to CDC.

primarily acute (sudden) infectious diseases, although some chronic and noninfectious diseases are reportable in some states. Health agencies at the local, state, and national levels routinely use the reported data for public health surveillance.

Laboratory Data. Laboratory reports form the basis of surveillance for selected diseases, including many viral illnesses and those caused by enteric pathogens such as salmonella and shigella. Laboratory reports may or may not be part of the notifiable disease reporting system.

Hospital Data. Almost all hospitals have computerized discharge records, primarily for financial and record-keeping purposes. These records typically include demographic data, diagnoses, operative procedures, length of stay, and costs, but exclude names, addresses, and other information that could identify individuals.

Several sources provide hospital discharge data on a national level. For example, one may obtain annual data on a national random sample of hospital records from the National Hospital Discharge Survey conducted by the NCHS. In addition, one can get data on Medicare inpatient and outpatient visits from the Health Care Financing Administration for Medicare recipients. Also, statewide and national surveillance systems collect data from samples of hospitals for a variety of specific health events. These include systems for the surveillance of birth defects, **nosocomial infections**, injuries, and drug-related emergency room visits.

Outpatient Health Care Data.   Although France has developed an extensive computerized surveillance system for outpatient data from physicians' offices, there is no comprehensive, timely outpatient surveillance system in the United States. At the local or state level, one may be able to obtain outpatient data from some physicians and health maintenance organizations that have computerized their medical records. At the national level, outpatient data can be obtained from the National Ambulatory Medical Care Survey, which is conducted periodically by NCHS, and from the commercial National Drug and Therapeutic Index. Both are random samples, from office-based physicians, of diagnostic, specialty, therapeutic, and disposition data. Finally, outpatient data are available from a network of interested family practice physicians, who report on a few selected health problems, including influenza-like illnesses.

Special Topics.   The majority of states now have some form of cancer registry. Many of these registries are part of the Surveillance, Epidemiology, and End Results (SEER) system supported by the National Cancer Institute. Each SEER Center attempts to identify every patient diagnosed with cancer in a designated geographical area (usually a state or large metropolitan area). For each patient, the SEER Center collects relevant demographic data as well as details on the type, site, and treatment of the cancer.

The post-marketing surveillance of adverse drug reactions and other adverse health events, in order to detect potential safety problems of marketed drugs, is the responsibility of the Food and Drug Administration (FDA). Each year, over ten-thousand reports of adverse events are submitted to the FDA by health care providers and pharmaceutical manufacturers.

In recent years, injury surveillance systems have increased. A number of systems in different jurisdictions now collect information on different types of injuries. At the national level, the National Highway Traffic Safety Administration collects information on fatal crashes occurring on public roadways.

Occupational illness is another area of current expansion. Surveillance data for occupational lead poisoning, pneumoconioses, and other occupationally related illnesses is collected in a growing number of states. Several states and the CDCP are also working to reestablish surveillance for elevated blood lead levels in children.

Surveys of Health and General Populations

All surveillance systems we have described collect data on the occurrence of some type of disease or other adverse health condition. Some systems, however, have been established to sample the health status of citizens in the community. For example, the NCHS periodically conducts the National Health and Nutrition Examination Survey (NHANES). In this survey, the NCHS examines a random sample of the U.S. population and

Nosocomial infections–infections that occur in an institutional setting, such as a hospital, skilled nursing facility, or a convalescent home.

records clinical examination and laboratory data, as well as demographic and medical history information. The NCHS has conducted this survey three times since 1960.

The NCHS also conducts the Health Interview Survey, which collects information on illness, disability, health service utilization, and activity restriction from a continuous sampling of over forty-thousand civilian households.

Finally, most health departments participate in the Behavioral Risk Factor Surveillance System in collaboration with the CDCP. This surveillance system uses telephone interviewers to collect information on smoking, alcohol use, seat-belt use, hypertension, weight, and other factors that affect health.

Surveillance Systems of Disease Indicators

Still other surveillance systems collect data on indicators of disease or of disease potential. These systems fall into four categories: animal populations, environmental data, drug/biological utilization, and student and employee data. Of these categories, the animal and environmental systems act as early-warning systems of disease potential. The other two categories collect disease-indicator data, which are more accessible than data on the particular diseases themselves.

Animal Populations. Monitoring animal populations is an important part of the surveillance system for certain diseases. Animal surveillance may include detecting and measuring the following kinds of information:

1. Animal morbidity and mortality caused by a disease that can affect humans (e.g., rabies)
2. The presence of a disease agent in wild and domestic sentinel animals (e.g., a survey of rodents for plague, of chickens for St. Louis encephalitis)
3. Changes in the size and distribution of the animal reservoirs and vectors of a disease (e.g., monitoring deer and ticks, which are hosts for the agent that causes Lyme disease)

Environmental Data. Public health agencies conduct routine environmental surveillance at the community level to detect the contamination of public water, milk, and food supplies. Agencies may also use environmental surveillance to focus on conditions in nature that support animal populations that may be reservoirs or vectors of disease. For example, agencies may monitor tire dumps and other potential breeding sites for mosquitoes. Other types of environmental surveillance have become important in recent years, such as environmental monitoring for radiation. In the workplace, "hazard surveillance," such as monitoring potentially harmful chemical, biological, and physical agents, can help in devising strategies for preventing illness and injury. Reports of environmental surveillance may often be obtained from local and state health departments.

Drug/Biological Utilization. State health departments and the CDCP are the only sources for a number of biologicals and drugs (e.g., botulism antitoxin, diphtheria antitoxin, and, until 1983, the anti-pneumocystis drug, pentamidine). By monitoring requests for these controlled biologicals, state health departments and the CDCP have an effective surveillance system for the diseases or exposures that these materials treat. Indeed, the CDCP noted an upsurge in pentamidine requests in 1981. This observation quickly led to the recognition of a nationwide epidemic of a disease soon to be named acquired immunodeficiency syndrome (AIDS).

Student and Employee Data. Public health agencies routinely use school absenteeism records to assess the pervasiveness of influenza-like illnesses in a community. Employee records, workers' compensation claims, and other occupational data are increasingly being used for the surveillance of occupational illness and injuries (Centers for Disease Control 1992).

Types of Measurement

The absolute numbers of events of illness and death are the primary data in epidemiology. Besides being the basic facts, their relative magnitude is also important. In a small community, the difference between two and twenty cases of a food poisoning outbreak would obviously be significant. While the absolute number of events is the first information needed to describe the distribution of illness and death in a population, there are two other parameters essential for analysis: (1) the population at risk of the events and (2) the relative impact of the events on the population at risk.

The **population at risk** is all the people exposed to the events of illness or death—all the individuals who could have become ill or died. Determining the population at risk is rarely simple and in practice an estimate is used. In "closed" populations, such as a school or factory, the population at risk of becoming ill can be determined accurately. But most populations of concern to epidemiology, such as in counties, cities, or states, are only counted at intervals of five or ten years in a population census. Between times, there are changes due to births, deaths, and migration. In this sense, they are "open" populations. In practice, the population at risk is estimated using the latest census figures. For example, for 1990, the population estimate for July 1 would be used as an estimate of the population at risk for the entire year.

The relationship between the events of illness or death and the population at risk in which they occur can be expressed as a rate, with the events being the numerator and the population at risk the denominator:

$$\text{Rate} = \frac{\text{Number of events}}{\text{Population at risk}} \times k$$

where *k* is a base constant, the most commonly used values being 100 (percent), 1,000, 10,000, and 100,000.

Population at risk–the population exposed to the risk of illness or death. In practice, it is difficult to determine the exact number of people who are exposed to factors that increase or decrease the risk of illness or death. Close approximations can be made with special populations, such as the numbers of workers in a factory, patrons of a restaurant, or children in a school.

The rate is always expressed as "per 1,000 or 10,000, etc. population," in a specified place and time. For example, if there were 50 deaths from influenza in a town called Rockton in 1990, which had a population in mid-1990 of 110,000, the rate would be calculated as follows:

$$\frac{50}{110,000} \times 100,000 = (0.000454)(100,000)$$

$$= 45.4 \text{ per } 100,000 \text{ population, Rockton, } 1990.$$

By convention, unless other units of time are specified, such as days or weeks, the rates are assumed to apply to units of years. Rates are relative numbers, relative to their denominator, and have the advantage of comparability. Rates of illness or death in populations can be compared between different time periods or between different places.

Rates of Illness

The most widely used measures of illness in a population are **incidence rates** and **prevalence rates**. Incidence is the number of *new* cases or events of a specified illness diagnosed or reported during a defined period of time. The incidence rate relates the number of cases to the number of persons in a particular population in which the cases occurred:

$$\text{Incidence rate} = \frac{\text{Number of new cases of an illness in a specified time}}{\text{Population at midpoint of the time period}} \times k$$

Incidence is the most important parameter in epidemiology. It tells us when new cases of a particular illness actually occur in time, and the incidence rate tells us the velocity of that illness in the population. Without this knowledge, we cannot directly associate the events of an illness with possible causal factors, or measure the relative importance of one illness over another.

Prevalence is the current number of cases, new and continuing, of a specified illness prevailing in a population. If this is determined for a particular point in time, it is called *point prevalence*, and if it is determined for a particular period of time, it is called *period prevalence*. The prevalence rate can be shown as follows:

$$\text{Prevalence rate} = \frac{\text{Number of current cases of an illness in a specified time period}}{\text{Population at midpoint of the time period}} \times k$$

Prevalence is not as useful as incidence in epidemiology, because it cannot specify exactly when cases of an illness took place and therefore relate them to possible causal factors. It is, however, an important indicator of the number of cases of illness that burden a population at one time, which is useful information for planning medical and other services. For some types of illness, such as most mental illnesses, prevalence is the only information we have. Incidence cannot be compiled because we do not

Incidence rate–the rate of new cases in a particular population for a specified period of time, where the numerator is the number of new cases of a specified illness diagnosed or reported during the specified time period, and the denominator is the population at the midpoint of the time period.

Prevalence rate–the rate of current (new and continuing) cases of an illness in a particular population for a specified period of time, where the numerator is the number of current cases of a specified illness diagnosed or reported during the specified time period, and the denominator is the population at midpoint of the time period. Prevalence at one point in time is called *point prevalence* and for a period of time is called *period prevalence.*

know with certainty when a case of mental illness begins. When both incidence and prevalence are available, we can make epidemiological comparisons. For example, the prevalence of arthritis (a long-term chronic disease of low death rate) in a population in one year will be much greater than the incidence, because of the accumulation of cases from year to year. The incidence of a short-term infectious disease, such as chicken pox, is likely to be high at certain times and low at others, and prevalence at any one time will reflect this incidence. Other special morbidity rates that are used in infectious disease epidemiology are given in Table 6.2.

Rates of Death

Death rates are important in epidemiology because they indicate the impact on a population of particular causes of death. Death rates can also

---

TABLE 6.2 Measures of Morbidity and Mortality

Morbidity Rates

Incidence rate
$$\frac{\text{Number of new cases of an illness in a specified time}}{\text{Population at midpoint of the time period}} \times k$$

Prevalence rate
$$\frac{\text{Number of current cases of an illness in a specified time period}}{\text{Population at midpoint of the time period}} \times k$$

Attack or case rate
An incidence rate for particular groups over short periods of time, usually expressed as a percentage.

Infection rate
$$\frac{\text{Number of all known infections, manifest and inapparent, in a specified time period}}{\text{Population at midpoint of the time period}} \times k$$

Fatality rate
$$\frac{\text{Number of deaths from a specified illness in a specified time period}}{\text{Number of cases of the specified illness in the specified time period}} \times k$$

Mortality Rates

Crude death rate
$$\frac{\text{Number of deaths in a specified time period}}{\text{Population at midpoint of the time period}} \times k$$

Age-specific death rate
$$\frac{\text{Number of deaths in a specified age group in a specified time period}}{\text{Population in the specified age group at midpoint of the time period}} \times k$$

Cause of death rate
$$\frac{\text{Number of deaths from a specified cause in a specified time period}}{\text{Population at midpoint of the time period}} \times k$$

TABLE 6.2 Measures of Morbidity and Mortality—cont'd

Infant and Maternal Mortality Rates

Infant death rate

$$\frac{\text{Number of deaths under 1 year of age in a specified time period}}{\text{Number of live births in the specified time}} \times k$$

Maternal death rate

$$\frac{\text{Number of deaths from pregnancy - related causes in a specified time period}}{\text{Number of live births in the specified time}} \times k$$

Neonatal death rate

$$\frac{\text{Number of deaths of infants under 28 days of age in a specified time period}}{\text{Number of live births in the specified time}} \times k$$

Perinatal death rate

$$\frac{\text{Number of fetal deaths of 28 or more weeks of gestation plus infant deaths under 7 days of age in a specified time period}}{\text{Number of live births and fetal deaths in the specified time period}} \times k$$

Post-neonatal death rate

$$\frac{\text{Number of infants dying between 28 days of age and the first year of life in a specified time period}}{\text{Number of live births in the specified time}} \times k$$

Fetal death rate

$$\frac{\text{Number of fetal deaths of 28 or more weeks of gestation in a specified time period}}{\text{Number of fetal deaths of 28 weeks or more of gestation plus live births in the specified time period}} \times k$$

Note: Most morbidity rates use a value of *k* of 1,000 or 10,000; mortality rates 1,000, 10,000 or 100,000; and infant and maternal mortality rates 1,000.

be used to study the association of disease with causal factors, although not as effectively as incidence rates. Because the mortality information needed for calculating death rates is more readily available than the morbidity information needed for incidence rates, death rates are often the only data available on the occurrence of disease.

A death rate expresses the relationship between population dying, population living, and time. In a population of 1,000 people who were alive at the beginning of a year, some will die throughout the year, some will be born, some will move in, and some will move away. At the end of the year, there may be more or less than 1,000 alive in the population, depending on the numbers of births, deaths, and migrants. The population living throughout the year can be thought of as a "year of life," some persons living a full year and others part of a year. The sum of all the full and part life years is the true population at risk of death during the year. In the example, if there were 150 deaths among the population during the year, and the life years summed to 900, the true rate of death during the year would be as follows:

$$\text{Death rate} = \frac{\text{Number of deaths in a specified time}}{\text{Population at risk (years of life)}} \times k$$

$$= \frac{150}{900} \times 1,000 = 166 \text{ per } 1,000 \text{ population}$$

In reality, it is impractical to compute the population at risk in terms of years of life lived for real populations. This can be done for hypothetical populations, as in the computation of a **life table**. For real populations the census count, or its estimate, for the midpoint of the time period is used. Death rates using this estimated population at risk are called **crude rates**.

The most commonly used measures of death in a population are the *crude* or *general death rate* and the *age-specific death rate*. These are usually reported for males and females separately. They can be calculated as shown:

$$\text{Crude death rate} = \frac{\begin{array}{c}\text{Number of deaths in a specified}\\ \text{time period}\end{array}}{\begin{array}{c}\text{Population at midpoint}\\ \text{of the time period}\end{array}} \times k$$

$$\text{Age specific death rate} = \frac{\begin{array}{c}\text{Number of deaths in a specified age}\\ \text{group in a specified time period}\end{array}}{\begin{array}{c}\text{Population in the specified age group}\\ \text{at midpoint of the time period}\end{array}} \times k$$

where k is usually 100,000.

Age-specific rates can be computed for illness events as well as for deaths. They show the impact of illness or death on each age group in a population, which is important because age itself is a major risk factor in many illnesses and in death. Figure 6.1 shows age-specific death rates in the United States for males and females from 1950 to 1990. Note that the highest rates occur among the oldest age group, but the lowest rates are among the 5–14 years age group. The under 1 year group has a comparatively high rate of death, reflecting the higher risks associated with the time around birth.

A comparison of male and female rates reveals that except for the 85 years and older age group, females have lower death rates than males in all age groups. Note too that the X axis of the chart uses a logarithmic scale to plot the rates. This is the correct scale to display rates and other relative numbers when proportions need to be constant. For example, if two different rates, one at 200 per 100,000 and the other at 2,000 per 100,000, are increasing at the same velocity, you want this to be shown correctly on the chart. A logarithmic scale will accomplish this because the proportions are the same—the distance between 20 and 40 on the scale is the same as between 200 and 400, and between 2,000 and 4,000.

Other kinds of mortality rates are given in Table 6.2. Note that infant and maternal death rates use special denominators.

The leading causes of death in a population are essential information for epidemiological research, health and medical services planning,

Life table–more accurately called a *mortality table*, it shows the percentage of persons who die at any given age. It is compiled from the history of mortality experience in a particular population. The table can be used to compute years of life lived, numbers surviving, and life expectancy at each age.

Crude rate–the general death rate in a particular population for a specified time period (usually one year), where the numerator is the total number of deaths occurring in the time period, and the denominator is the population at the midpoint of the time period. It is called "crude" because the denominator is an estimate of the years of life lived by the population at risk of death.

FIGURE 6.1

Age- and Sex-Specific
Death Rates, United
States, 1950–1990.

Source: National Center for
Health Statistics. *Monthly
vital statistics report:
Advance report of final
mortality statistics, 1989.*
Vol. 41, No. 7, January 7,
1993, Hyattsville, MD.

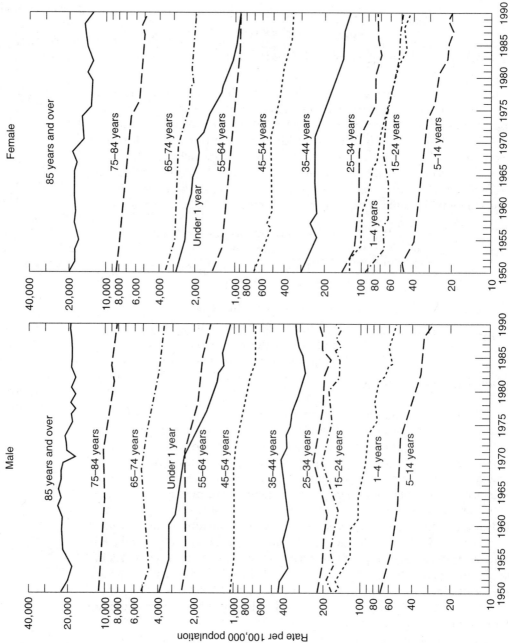

and health education. These are indicated by cause of death rates, as shown here:

$$\text{Cause of death rate} = \frac{\begin{array}{c}\text{Number of deaths from a specified cause}\\\text{in a specified time period}\end{array}}{\text{Population at midpoint of the time period}} \times k$$

where k is usually $100,000$.

Percentages are also used to show the proportion of deaths due to each cause. The leading causes of death for the United States, by major age groups, are shown in Table 6.3.

The Adjustment of Rates

Rates are affected by population characteristics, such as age, sex, ethnicity, and occupation, and by the way the event (for instance, an infectious disease), behaves in the host population. Crude rates are the actual rates of illness or death in a population, and they include all the variables that can influence the rate. In epidemiology, we often want to control known variables, such as sex and age, so that the resultant rates will more closely reflect the impact of other variables in the causal process. For example, the death rate from cancer of the breast in the United States in 1989 was 17.4 per 100,000 population. Knowing that this disease is much more common in women than in men, we would probably want to adjust or control for sex. The rates by sex are, respectively, 33.7 and 0.2 per 100,000 population—over 168 times more frequent in women than in men.

Age-Adjusted Rates

Differences in the age structure of populations over time (such as Illinois in 1960 compared to 1990) or between states (for instance, Hawaii and Vermont in 1990) can have a strong influence on the frequency of crude rates. The crude death rates for Illinois in 1960 were less than those in 1990, in large part because the population was younger in 1960 and there were fewer older people dying. Similarly, in 1990, Hawaii had a lower crude rate of death than Vermont because it had a more youthful population. As mentioned earlier in this chapter, age-specific rates are one way to adjust or control for age effects. However, there are situations in which a single rate for the total population is more useful for comparative purposes, such as comparing death rates among the fifty U.S. states.

A single age-adjusted rate for the total population is calculated using a standard population, or standard illness or death rates. For example, the U.S. population for 1940 is used as the standard for computing age-adjusted rates for states by the National Center for Health Statistics (Figure 6.2). There are two methods of calculating age-adjusted rates; the *direct* method uses a standard population, and the *indirect* method uses a standard set of illness or death rates. The computation of age-adjusted rates using these methods is shown in Figure 6.3.

TABLE 6.3 Deaths and Death Rates for the Ten Leading Causes of Death in Specified Age Groups, United States, 1991 (Rates per 100,000 Population)

Rank Order[1]	Cause of Death and Age (Ninth Revision International Classification of Disease, 1975)	Number	Rate
	All races*, both sexes		
	1–4 years		
	All causes	7,214	47.4
1	Accidents and adverse effects........E800-E949	2,665	17.5
...	Motor vehicle accidents..........E810-E825	902	5.9
...	All other accidents and adverse effects........E800-E807, E826-E949	1,763	11.6
2	Congenital anomalies..........740-759	871	5.7
3	Malignant neoplasms, including neoplasms of lymphatic and hematopoietic tissues..140-208	526	3.5
4	Homicide and legal intervention......E960-E978	428	2.8
5	Diseases of heart.........390-398, 402, 404-429	332	2.2
6	Pneumonia and influenza..........480-487	207	1.4
7	Human immunodeficiency virus infection..........*042-044	155	1.0
8	Certain conditions originating in the perinatal period..........760-779	140	0.9
9	Septicemia..........038	91	0.6
10	Benign neoplasms, carcinoma in situ, and neoplasms of uncertain behavior and of unspecified nature..........210-239	76	0.5
...	All other causes..........Residual	1,723	11.3
	All races*, both sexes		
	5–14 years		
	All causes	8,479	23.6
1	Accidents and adverse effects........E800-E949	3,660	10.2
...	Motor vehicle accidents..........E810-E825	2,011	5.6
...	All other accidents and adverse effects........E800-E807, E826-E949	1,649	4.6
2	Malignant neoplasms, including neoplasms of lymphatic and hematopoietic tissues..140-208	1,106	3.1
3	Homicide and legal intervention......E960-E978	519	1.4
4	Congenital anomalies..........740-759	487	1.4
5	Diseases of heart.........390-398, 402, 404-429	281	0.8
6	Suicide..........E950-E959	266	0.7
7	Pneumonia and influenza..........480-487	135	0.4

Rank Order[1]	Cause of Death and Age (Ninth Revision International Classification of Diseases, 1975)	Number	Rate
8	Chronic obstructive pulmonary disease and allied conditions..........490-496	122	0.3
9	Human immunodeficiency virus infection..........*042-044	104	0.3
10	Cerebrovascular diseases..........430-438	86	0.2
...	All other causes..........Residual	1,713	4.8
	All races, both sexes		
	15–24 years		
...	All causes	36,452	100.1
1	Accidents and adverse effects........E800-E949	15,278	42.0
...	Motor vehicle accidents..........E810-E825	11,664	32.0
...	All other accidents and adverse effects........E800-E807, E826-E949	3,614	9.9
2	Homicide and legal intervention......E960-E978	8,159	22.4
3	Suicide..........E950-E959	4,751	13.1
4	Malignant neoplasms, including neoplasms of lymphatic and hematopoietic tissues..........140-208	1,814	5.0
5	Diseases of heart.........390-398, 402, 404-429	990	2.7
6	Human immunodeficiency virus infection..........*042-044	613	1.7
7	Congenital anomalies..........740-759	449	1.2
8	Pneumonia and influenza..........480-487	256	0.7
9	Cerebrovascular diseases..........430-438	219	0.6
10	Chronic obstructive pulmonary diseases and allied conditions..........490-496	209	0.6
...	All other causes..........Residual	3,714	10.2
	All races*, both sexes		
	25–44 years		
...	All causes	147,750	179.9
1	Accidents and adverse effects........E800-E949	26,526	32.3
...	Motor vehicle accidents..........E810-E825	15,082	18.4
...	All other accidents and adverse effects........E800-E807, E826-E949	11,444	13.9

TABLE 6.3 Deaths and Death Rates for the Ten Leading Causes of Death in Specified Age Groups, United States, 1991 (Rates per 100,000 Population)—cont'd

Rank Order[1]	Cause of Death and Age (Ninth Revision International Classification of Disease, 1975)	Number	Rate
2	Malignant neoplasms, including neoplasms of lymphatic and hematopoietic tissues....140-208	22,228	27.1
3	Human immunodeficiency virus infection....042*-044*	21,747	26.5
4	Diseases of heart....390-398, 402, 404-429	15,822	19.3
5	Homicide and legal intervention....E960-E978	12,372	15.1
6	Suicide....E950-E959	12,281	14.9
7	Chronic liver disease and cirrhosis....571	4,449	5.4
8	Cerebrovascular diseases....433-438	3,343	4.1
9	Diabetes melitus....250	2,211	2.7
10	Pneumonia and influenza....480-487	2,203	2.7
...	All other causes....Residual	24,568	29.9
	All races*, both sexes 45-64 years		
...	All causes	368,754	788.9
1	Malignant neoplasms, including neoplasms of lymphatic and hematopoietic tissues....140-208	134,117	286.9
2	Diseases of heart....390-398, 402, 404-429	105,359	225.4
3	Cerebrovascular diseases....430-438	14,464	30.9
4	Accidents and adverse effects....E800-E949	13,693	29.3
	Motor vehicle accidents....E810-E825	6,616	14.2
...	All other accidents and adverse effects....E800-E807, E826-E949	7,077	15.1
5	Chronic obstructive pulmonary diseases and allied conditions....490-496	12,769	27.3
6	Chronic liver disease and cirrhosis....571	10,497	22.5
7	Diabetes melitus....250	10,045	21.5
8	Suicide....E950-E959	7,224	15.5
9	Human immunodeficiency virus infection....*042-*044	6,286	13.4
10	Pneumonia and influenza....480-487	5,476	11.7
...	All other causes....Residual	48,824	104.4
	All races*, both sexes 65 years and over		
...	All causes	1,563,527	4,924.0
1	Diseases of heart....390-398, 402, 404-429	597,267	1,831.0
2	Malignant neoplasms, including neoplasms of lymphatic and hematopoietic tissues....140-208	354,768	1,117.3
3	Cerebrovascular diseases....430-438	125,139	334.1
4	Chronic obstructive pulmonary diseases and allied conditions....490-496	76,412	240.6
5	Pneumonia and influenza....480-487	68,962	217.2
6	Diabetes melitus....250	36,528	115.0
7	Accidents and adverse effects....E800-E949	26,444	83.3
	Motor vehicle accidents....E810-E825	7,044	22.2
...	All other accidents and adverse effects....E800-E807, E826-E949	19,400	61.1
8	Nephritis, nephrotic syndrome, and nephrosis....580-589	17,963	56.6
9	Atherosclerosis....440	16,568	52.2
10	Septicemia....038	15,888	50.0
...	All other causes....Residual	227,588	716.7

Source: Data from National Center for Health Statistics. Aug. 31, 1993. *Monthly vital statistics report: Advance report of final mortality statistics, 1989.* Vol. 42, No. 2. Hyattsville, MD: NCHS.

FIGURE 6.2
Crude and Age-Adjusted
Death Rates, United
States, 1940–1989.

Source: National Center for
Health Statistics. *Monthly
vital statistics report:
Advance report of final mortality statistics, 1989.* Vol.
40, No. 8, January 7, 1992,
Hyattsville, MD.

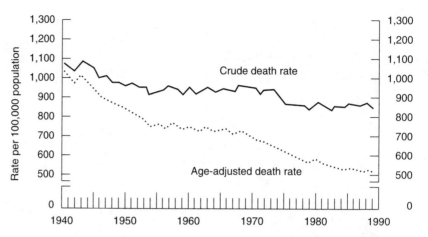

*Age-adjusted by the direct method using the U.S. population of 1940
as standard.

FIGURE 6.3
Computation of Age-
Adjusted Rates.

In 1980, there were 228 deaths from cancer of the lung in the resident population of Honolulu City and County in
Hawaii. The population in mid-1980 was 762,565, giving a crude rate of 29.9 per 100,000 population. In 1980, the
crude rate for the United States for cancer of the lung was 47.9 per 100,000 population. In order to control for age
effects on these crude rates, age-adjusted rates can be computed by the direct or the indirect method.

Direct Method

Age Group Years* x	Honolulu County, 1980			United States, 1980	
	Popn. nPx	Lung Cancer Deaths nDx	Death Rates nMx	Standard Population nP^{s}x	Expected Deaths (nMx)(nP^{s}x)
< 24	334,539	0	– – –	93,777,167	– – –
25–44	232,786	6	.0000257	62,716,549	1,612
45–64	139,872	93	.0006648	44,502,662	29,585
65–84	51,360	114	.0022196	23,309,360	51,737
85 +	4,008	15	.0037425	2,240,067	8,383
Total	762,565	228	– – –	226,545,805	91,317

$$\text{Age-adjusted rate} = \frac{\sum \left(nMx \right)\left(nP_x^s \right)}{\sum nP_x^s}$$
(direct method)

$$= \frac{\text{Expected deaths}}{\text{Standard Population}} = \frac{91,317}{226,545,805}$$

$$= 40.3 \text{ per } 100,000 \text{ population}$$

Measurement of Illness and Death

FIGURE 6.3 CONT'D

Indirect Method

Age Group Years* x	United States, 1980			Honolulu County, 1980	
	Standard Population nPx	Lung Cancer Deaths D	Death Rate nMx	Population nPx	Expected Deaths (nMx)(nPx)
< 24	93,777,167	88	.0000009	334,539	0
25–44	62,716,549	2,756	.0000439	232,786	10
45–64	44,502,662	45,215	.0010160	139,872	142
65–84	23,309,360	57,304	.0024584	51,360	126
85 +	2,240,067	4,134	.0018455	4,008	7
Total	226,545,805	109,497	– – –	762,565	285

$$\text{Age-adjusted rate} = \left[\frac{D}{\Sigma\left(nM_x^s\right)(nPx)}\right]\left[\frac{\Sigma\left(nM_x^s\right)\left(nP_x^s\right)}{\Sigma nP_x^s}\right]$$
(indirect method)

$$= \left[\frac{\text{Observed deaths}}{\text{Expected deaths}}\right]\left[\begin{array}{l}\text{Crude rate in the}\\ \text{standard popula}\end{array}\right.$$

$$= \left[\frac{228}{285}\right][.0004789]$$

$$= 38.3 \text{ per } 100,000 \text{ population}$$

Standardized Mortality Ratio

$$\text{SMR} = \left[\frac{\text{Observed deaths}}{\text{Expected deaths}}\right][100]$$

$$= \left[\frac{228}{285}\right][100] = 80\%$$

Notation D = Number of deaths or cases for a specified population.

nPx = The number of persons at age x for a specified population midpoint in the time period.

nMx = The mortality or morbidity rate at age x for a specified population and time period.

s = Standard population.

*In practice, many more age groups are used than the five shown here which are only to illustrate the method. Usually ages are grouped by five years to give 18 to 20 groups. Rate computation is then much more sensitive to differences between age groups.

Both direct and indirect methods have practical and theoretical importance. In practice, the direct method cannot always be employed, because mortality or morbidity data by age group are not always available for counties or other small administrative units of interest. Even when such data are available, the numbers may be too small to compute reliable rates. In theory, the direct method is preferable when comparing total death rates, or rates for one cause of death, because with this method the population is standard or held constant. Also, rates that have been adjusted by the direct method can be directly compared to one another. For example, using a standard population and adjusting the rates for several states (such as Illinois, Arizona, and Hawaii), we can compare the adjusted rates across all states. With the indirect method, multiple rates cannot be compared. Only the adjusted rate can be compared with the standard rate for an observed or expected ratio. The indirect method is preferable when comparing rates for different causes of death or illness in the same population, because with this method the mortality or morbidity experience is standard. All age-adjusted rates are abstractions and cannot be compared with crude rates. Nor can rates that have been age-adjusted by the direct method be compared with those that have been adjusted by the indirect method (Ferrara 1980; Dever 1984).

Standardized Mortality (or Morbidity) Ratio

A variation of the age-adjusted rate by the indirect method is the standardized mortality or morbidity ratio (SMR), which has been widely used in Canada and in European countries. It expresses the relative proportion of illness or death as a percentage, where 100 is the standard population average. An SMR of 95 represents a rate that is 5 percent less than the standard, and an SMR of 110 would be 10 percent above. The SMR is often used in mapping mortality or morbidity distributions.

Other Measurements and Issues

Life Expectancy

Life expectancy at birth, or later ages, is used for national and international comparisons to indicate health change in populations over time. In 1950, many less-developed countries had population life expectancies at birth of 25 years. In 1991, no country had a life expectancy of less than 40 years, indicating considerable improvement, principally in reduction of mortality in the first five years of life. There continue to be marked variations between countries all over the world (Table 6.4).

Years of Potential Life Lost

This measure is used to show the importance of certain causes of death in reducing life expectancy, especially in the adolescent and younger adult years. It focuses on the age groups up to 65 years and computes the years of life lost due to various causes of death. For example, if a person aged 20 years dies from AIDS, society has lost 65 − 20 = 45 potential life years. Using this measure, it can be demonstrated that deaths due to unintentional (accidental) injuries (especially in motor-vehicle crashes), cancers (especially cancer of the lung), suicides and homicides, diseases of the

TABLE 6.4 Life Expectancy at Birth, Selected Countries, 1991

Country	Life Expectancy in Years at Birth
Japan	79
Sweden	78
France	77
Canada	77
Hong Kong	77
Australia	76
Cuba	76
Israel	76
United Kingdom	75
United States	75
Singapore	75
Chile	72
Poland	72
Jordan	70
Russia	70
Mexico	70
China	69
Iran	65
Brazil	65
Philippines	64
Kenya	63
Indonesia	61
India	57
Papua-New Guinea	54
Bangladesh	53
Haiti	53
Nepal	52
Nigeria	48
Ethiopia	46
Sierra Leone	42
Afghanistan	41

Source: Data from Population Reference Bureau. 1991. Washington, D.C.: Government Printing Office.

heart, congenital anomalies, and human immunodeficiency virus infections are currently the most significant in the United States in causing early death and lost years of life (Table 6.5).

Risk

Risk is the chance or probability of something happening, and in epidemiology it is the probability of illness or death. The risk of death or illness is technically not the same as the rate of death or illness, although the terms risk and rate are commonly used interchangeably. Earlier we defined the true rate of dying in a population during a year as the ratio between the number of deaths and the population at risk, or "years of

TABLE 6.5 Years of Potential Life Lost Before Age 65 and Death Rates, by Cause of Death, United States, 1990

Cause of Death	Potential Years of Life Lost*	Cause-Specific Crude Death Rate per 100,000
ALL CAUSES	12,083,228	861.9
Unintentional injuries	2,147,094	37.3
Cancers	1,839,900	201.7
Suicides and homicides	1,520,780	22.5
Diseases of heart	1,349,027	289.0
Congenital anomalies	644,651	5.3
Human immunodeficiency virus infection	644,245	9.6
Prematurity	415,638	2.5
Sudden infant death syndrome	347,713	2.2

Source: Data from National Center for Health Statistics. May 8, 1992. *Morbidity and mortality weekly report.* Vol. 41, p. 314. Hyattsville, MD: NCHS.

*Total years of potential life lost are estimated for persons between birth and 65 years of age at the time of death and are derived from the product of the number of deaths in each age category and the difference between 65 years and the age at the midpoint of each category.

Risk–the chance or probability of an event happening in a population. In epidemiology, it is the chance of an illness or death in a population. Risk applies to populations, not to individuals. The risk of a particular person dying this year is unknown; the risk of persons in a particular age group dying this year is known from what has happened in past years.

life." In the example of a population of 1,000 persons, there were 150 deaths during the year, and the rate was 150/900 (life years) = 0.166, or 166.0 per 1,000 population. *Rate* here is the number of people who died during the time period divided by the number of years of life, or the number of people alive during the time period and at risk of dying. In contrast, the risk of dying during the year would be 150/1,000 = 0.15, or 15 percent. **Risk** here is the number of people who died during the time period divided by the number of people at the beginning of the time period who were at risk. Risk is usually expressed as a probability or ratio, not as a rate per population. Other special applications of risk, such as relative risk and absolute risk, are discussed in Chapter 8.

Common Errors in Measurement

Rates and proportions are relative numbers and always require interpretation. The absolute numbers from which the rates are derived should always be reported. For instance, if a local health department announced that it had helped reduce the frequency of motor-vehicle crashes in its community by 75 percent, we might be impressed until we learned that there were four crashes in one year and one the next. The absolute numbers are necessary to interpret the significance of the percentage. Rates and percentages based on small numbers of events in small populations are also subject to random statistical variation. In other words, the drop in the number of motor-vehicle crashes reported by the local health department might have been due to chance rather than to any public health intervention. The problem of small denominators in computing rates can be especially serious when data are broken down into various strata, for example, by age, sex, or diagnostic group. In these instances, the results may be meaningless.

Rates use different bases, and it is important to check what base is being used. In a percentage the base is 100, so a proportion of 2/80 would be (2/80)(100) = 2.5 percent. In a rate, the same proportion could be multiplied by 1,000, 10,000 or 100,000 to yield rates of 25, 250, and 2,500, respectively. It would be an error to compare percentages and rates that were using different bases.

The comparison of rates from the same population requires care. The events in the numerator may come from entirely different groups of individuals in the same population. For example, a high rate of liver disease and a high rate of alcoholism in a population might be thought to be generated by the same group of individuals. The group, however, may be only partially the same, or totally different. This requires further investigation, because the rates by themselves tell us nothing about whether or not the events in their numerators are associated. For a more detailed discussion of the methods of measurement in epidemiology see Kahn and Sempos (1989).

Summary

The epidemiological measurement of illness (morbidity) and deaths (mortality) in populations is done principally through rates, which relate the number of cases of illness or death (events), to the population in which the events occurred (the population at risk). Rates are expressed as per 1,000 or 10,000 or 100,000 population, in a specified time or place. The adjustment of rates by sex, age, ethnicity, or other population characteristics is important in order to control known variables, so that the impact of other variables is revealed. The risk of illness or death is the probability of these events occurring in a population. Risk is not the same as the rate of becoming ill or dying in a population through time.

Mortality and morbidity data can be obtained through published reports by the National Center for Health Statistics, the Centers for Disease Control and Prevention, and a variety of special reports from many different health and social organizations. Some data are routinely collected and other data such as those gathered in special surveys are often utilized for surveillance purposes.

Surveillance data involving animal and environmental systems are often collected to alert public health officials as to pending potential problems. Drug/biological and student/employee data are collected to alert officials to problems and to track occupational illnesses.

Discussion Questions

1. Assume that there were 60 new cases of asthma reported during a year in a population of 56,890. There were an additional 270 cases on record from previous years. What is (a) the prevalence rate and (b) the incidence rate of asthma in this population?

2. Given the following data, calculate the crude death rates per 100,000 population for Canada, Mexico, and the United States:

Country	Population	Deaths	Rate
Canada	26.6 million	0.19 million	
Mexico	88.6 million	0.52 million	
United States	251.4 million	2.24 million	

   Can you think of a reason why the rate for Mexico is less than that of Canada or the United States?

3. Describe the four major surveillance systems of disease or disease potential.

4. Explain the difference between a crude and an age-specific death rate.

5. Why are rates adjusted for age, sex, ethnicity, and occupation? Explain your reasoning.

6. What is the basic difference between a direct method of age adjustment and an indirect method? Of what practical and theoretical importance are they?

References

Benenson, A. S. 1990. *Control of communicable diseases in man.* 15th ed. Washington, D.C.: American Public Health Association.

Centers for Disease Control. 1992. *Principles of epidemiology.* Atlanta, GA: U.S. Department of Health and Human Services.

Dever, G. E. A. 1984. *Epidemiology in health services management.* Rockville, MD: Aspen Systems Corp.

Ferrara, C. P. 1980. *Vital and health statistics: Techniques of community health analysis.* Atlanta, GA: Centers for Disease Control.

Gittelsohn, A. M. 1982. On the distribution of underlying causes of death. *American Journal of Public Health* 72:133–140.

Gobbato, F., F. Vecchiet, D. Barbierato, M. Melato, and R. Manconi. 1982. Inaccuracy of death certificate diagnoses in malignancy: An analysis of 1,405 autopsied cases. *Human Pathology* 13:1036–1038.

Kahn, H. A., and C. T. Sempos. 1989. *Statistical methods in epidemiology.* New York: Oxford University Press.

World Health Organization. 1988. The surveillance of communicable diseases. *WHO Chronicle* 22:1,439–1,444.

CHAPTER 7

Descriptive Epidemiology

Introduction

In descriptive epidemiology, we organize and summarize data according to time, place, and person. These three characteristics are sometimes called the epidemiological variables.

Compiling and analyzing data by time (when), place (where) and person (who) are desirable for several reasons. First, the investigator becomes familiar with the basic data and with the scope of the public health problem under investigation. Second, this method provides an in-depth description of the health of a population that is easily communicated to other professionals and the lay public. Third, such an approach identifies the populations that are of greater risk of acquiring a particular disease. Thus, such information provides important clues to the causes of the disease, and these clues can then be formulated into testable hypotheses.

Time

Time can be divided into many subunits, such as minutes, hours, days, weeks, months, years, and decades, depending on the purpose and information desired by an epidemiologist. For example, in an outbreak of food-borne disease, hours or days are generally important in attempting to seek out the possible agent or source of contamination. A median incubation period of 12–14 hours may point to salmonella, or a period of 3–6 hours from ingestion of contaminated food to illness may reflect an outbreak of staphylococcus origin. When the time span exceeds one or several decades, however, problems may arise as to the comparability of data, because over time changes may occur in standards of diagnosis, reporting, and the definition of a case. Factors related to time that are of importance to epidemiology include secular trends, seasonal and cyclical variations, and point epidemics.

Secular Trends

Secular trends are long-term trends that usually involve examining disease rates over one or more decades. Some diseases may display a progressive increase, decrease, or a pattern of rising and falling rates over years or decades. For example, Figure 7.1 shows the secular trend of syphilis from 1956 to 1993. It should be noted that despite the publicity given to sexually transmitted diseases, syphilis has increased among both sexes from 1987 to 1990. On the other hand, rubeola (regular measles) has shown a dramatic decrease since the measles vaccine was licensed in 1963. However, periodic epidemics of measles still occur, even though state laws mandate that children be immunized before being admitted to school. Measles will be further discussed in this chapter in relation to age as an important variable in disease epidemiology.

Another example of a secular trend can be observed in Figure 7.2, which shows the *ectopic* (out of place) pregnancy death rates from 1970 to 1987. From 1970, when the Centers for Disease Control first began to initiate surveillance activities, until 1987, the rate of ectopic pregnancies increased nearly fourfold. Similarly, the rate of ectopic pregnancies per 1,000 live births rose approximately fivefold, and the rate per 10,000 females of reproductive age (15–44) increased about fivefold (Centers for Disease Control 1990). Chow (1990) cites that "such factors as heightened awareness among medical providers, improved diagnostic technology, and an increased occurrence of pelvic inflammatory disease resulting from sexually transmitted diseases may account for this dramatic increase." Fortunately, due to early detection and subsequent medical intervention, the overall case fatality rate declined during this time period.

FIGURE 7.1

Syphilis (Primary and Secondary)—By Sex, United States, 1956–1993.

Source: Summary of Notifiable Diseases, United States, 1991. *Morbidity and Mortality Weekly Report.* Centers for Disease Control, Atlanta, GA, October 21, 1994.

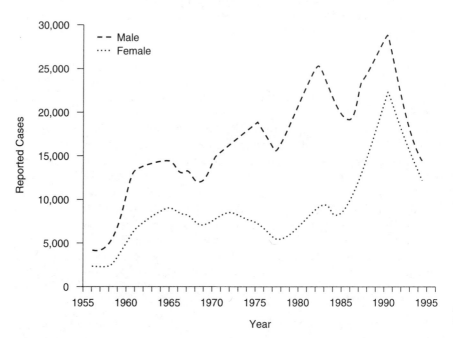

Descriptive Epidemiology

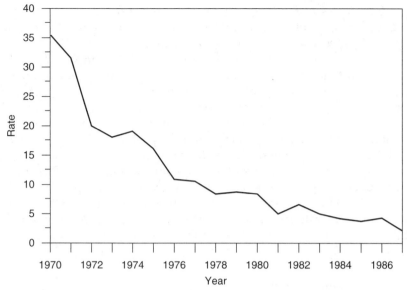

FIGURE 7.2
Ectopic Pregnancy
Death Rates,* by Year—
United States,
1970–1987.

Source: CDC, Ectopic
Pregnancy, United States,
1987. MMWR, 39:401–407,
1990.

*Per 10,000 ectopic pregnancies.

Secular trends for various diseases may be influenced by a number of factors. For example, certain viruses may alter their genetic structure, thereby negating prior immunity, such as in the case of influenza pandemics that appear to occur approximately every decade. Also, certain pathogens may become drug resistant to antibiotics, as is evident with drug-resistant cases of tuberculosis. Other factors may include improved diagnostic and treatment modalities, changing the case definitions for a given disease, and alterations in the physical, social, and cultural environments.

Seasonal and Cyclical Variations

Seasonal and cyclical variations involve diseases or accidents that often display regular recurring increases and decreases during a year, or over periods of several months or years. Some diseases will display annual or seasonal peaks, while others will occur in cycles of several years duration. For example, **zoonotic diseases** that rely on **arthropod** transmission increase or decrease in relation to seasonal variations in tick or other insect vectors. Normally, tick activity is abundant in the spring or early summer, thereby establishing a seasonal pattern for Rocky Mountain spotted fever and Lyme disease. Also, respiratory illnesses are less common in the summer months, due, in part, to schools being closed. Activities are more likely to occur outdoors, where airborne agents become greatly diluted. When schools reopen in the fall, however, a resurgence of respiratory disease occurs, with peaks of cases in September, midwinter and early spring.

Zoonotic diseases–infectious diseases transmissible under normal conditions from animals to humans.

Arthropod–any of a phylum of invertebrate animals with articulate (jointed) body and limbs, such as insects, arachnids, and crustaceans.

Regardless of the infecting agent or its source of origin, the proportion of susceptible persons in a population is an extremely important factor influencing the occurrence of a disease, especially with regard to agents that are transmitted person to person. For example, Fox (1970) has defined *herd immunity* as the "resistance of a group to invasion and spread of an infectious agent, based on the immunity of a high proportion of individual members of the group." Mausner and Kramer (1985) believe that herd immunity is an important factor that underscores the dynamics of **propagated** epidemics and the **periodicity** of disease, such as chicken pox and measles prior to the widespread use of vaccines. Therefore, during the course of an epidemic, a number of susceptible individuals contract the disease, thus providing multiple sources of infection to others. However, since the disease victims develop immunity as the epidemic progresses, the proportion of nonsusceptibles in the population increases and the size of the remaining susceptible population declines.

Propagated source epidemic–an epidemic in which infections are transmitted from person to person or animal to animal in such a fashion that cases identified cannot be attributed to agents transmitted from a single source.

Periodicity–recurring at intervals.

Point Epidemics

Point epidemics are short-term variations in excess disease or injury occurrence and can be commonly measured in days, weeks, or sometimes months. The most common examples of point epidemics are those that result from human ingestion of microbiologically contaminated food or water. Unless a relatively large number of persons are affected, as in schools, military groups, company conventions, or social gatherings, episodes of this nature often escape official public health attention.

Point epidemics generally indicate (1) that the affected persons were exposed to the same causal factor at approximately the same time; (2) that the disease is not readily spread by direct person-to-person contact; and (3) that the incubation period is of short duration.

Epidemics of infectious disease are generally self-limited, with the exception of the **continuing source** type of epidemic. Most often, the epidemic curve of disease occurrence displays the familiar bell-shaped curve of normal distribution. Therefore, the evaluation of epidemic control measures may be complicated by the knowledge that had no control efforts been undertaken, the disease would have eventually declined. It is difficult to determine whether or not sometimes a decline in an epidemic was caused by control efforts.

Continuing source epidemic–an epidemic in which there is a source that serves as a focal point for the continuing spread of the agent, e.g., contaminated well water.

Place

Place refers to a designated geographical area, such as latitude, longitude, nation, state, region, county, urban, rural, location of residence, institutional, noninstitutional, and so forth. Basically, the association of a disease with a place implies that the factors of greatest etiological importance are present either in the inhabitants, or in the environment, or both. According to Fox (1970), "true association with place is suggested when age adjusted risk of disease increases for immigrants and decreases for emigrants, when all ethnic groups present are at similar high risk and when similar ethnic groups residing elsewhere are at lower risk." It should be noted, though, that spurious or false associations of disease, illness, or injury with place may be the product of differences in the reliability and completeness of disease recognition and reporting, and the failure to adjust statistically for age-sex differences in population groups.

Variations in Rates Among Regions and Nations

Because of differences in the completeness of reporting and the reliability of data, caution must be observed in interpreting disease occurrence among nations. Information is routinely gathered and published by the World Health Organization for many countries in the world for notifiable disease and causes of death. However, variations between countries with regard to the availability, quality, and distribution of medical care may directly affect the reliability of diagnosis and the completeness of recording deaths and births. Generally, in newly developing nations, infant mortality rates may be somewhat unreliable, since reporting is often more complete for infant deaths than for births.

Substantial differences in the prevalence of disease often exist between nations, which may suggest some useful hypotheses about disease. One must keep in mind, though, that descriptive epidemiology may only suggest exploratory hypotheses. Nevertheless, descriptive data can often be of value to epidemiologists in generating hypotheses for further intensive study of causal factors.

For example, Hungary has the highest male age-adjusted death rate for all cancers, whereas Denmark has the highest rate for females. In contrast, Peru has the lowest cancer death rate for all sites of cancer for both sexes. With respect to lung cancer, Scotland has the highest age-adjusted rate for males, and Barbados has the highest rate for females. Such differences may suggest useful hypotheses for more vigorous testing. It is interesting to note that the lowest age-adjusted deaths from cancer of the stomach for both sexes occur in the United States, while the highest rates are found in Costa Rica for males and females combined, with Japan a close second. Interestingly, second-generation Japanese Americans who have moved to the United States have about the same risk as Americans for stomach cancer. This finding also correlates extremely well with breast cancer. Japan has the lowest mortality rate for cancer of the breast, and the United States has a rate approximately three times higher, but when Japanese women migrate to the United States, their rate after two generations approximates that of American females (Duncan 1988). One therefore might hypothesize that there are biological, social, physical, and medical differences in the environment between the two countries that may be worthy of intensive epidemiological research.

In comparing intranational rates (rates within regions of the same nation), a number of interesting comparisons have been observed. Multiple sclerosis is more prevalent in temperate climates, such as those found in northern Europe and the northern United States than in the tropics. Also, histoplasmosis (a fungus disease) tends to follow the tornado belt throughout the Ohio and Mississippi River valleys, where more than 80 percent of the adult population tests positive for presence of the organism (Norton 1987). It is widely believed that strong winds and tornadoes widely disseminate the fungus throughout the so-called "tornado valleys," where the organism thrives in humid climates. In the past decade, the isolation rates of salmonella enteritidis have increased dramatically in New England and, more recently, in the mid-Atlantic states. Contaminated food was implicated in 64 percent of the outbreaks. Consequently, health authorities have advised the public not to eat raw or undercooked eggs and to avoid eating food that contains raw eggs, such as Caesar salad and homemade eggnog or mayonnaise (Centers for Disease Control 1989).

Urban-Rural Comparisons

Infectious diseases generally spread more rapidly in urban areas than in rural areas, because of the greater population density and the greater opportunity for susceptible urban residents to come in contact with a source of infection. However, due to the great mobility of our population today, many of these differences have greatly narrowed. On the other hand, some zoonotic diseases that are transmitted from animals to humans, including vectorborne diseases, often have a greater incidence in rural areas. Such is the case for human plague that was reported in rural areas of the southwest, particularly in New Mexico, Arizona, California, and Colorado in 1988. Many of the human plague cases were among Native Americans. The risk factors for Native Americans included residence in plague foci and life-style (e.g., sheepherding, hunting of prairie dogs and rabbits, and residing in hogans that may attract rodents) (Centers for Disease Control 1988).

Any conclusions based on urban-rural differences should be approached with caution because of *confounding*, in which the influence of one exposure is mixed with the effect of another. For example, people who drink alcohol also are more apt to drink coffee. Thus, when a study is conducted to examine alcohol consumption and breast cancer, the possible confounding role of coffee and caffeine needs to be considered. In this case, the estimated effect of alcohol on breast cancer will be confounded by caffeine consumption, if caffeine and alcohol use are correlated and caffeine use independently influences the risk of breast cancer. It is also possible that more urban dwellers consume more coffee and have higher rates of smoking, which add to the confounding effect unless these potential confounders are controlled through appropriate study designs and statistical procedures.

Descriptive Epidemiology

Personal or Host Factors

Basic demographic and social characteristics of people or cohorts are of special concern to epidemiologists. The major characteristics studied include age, sex, race or ethnic group, social class, marital status, religion, occupation, life-style, nutrition, and immunization status. All of these host factors and perhaps others are important to the extent that they affect the risk of exposure to a source of infection and the host's resistance or susceptibility to infection, disease, and injury.

Host factors can be put in certain categories: (1) acquired or **inherent** characteristics, such as age, race, sex, and immunization and marital status; (2) activities, such as work, play, recreational pursuits, religious practices, and customs; or (3) the circumstances under which people live (social, economic, and environmental conditions). Generally, such characteristics aid in determining, to a large degree, which persons are at the greatest risk of acquiring infections or experiencing other undesirable illnesses or injuries.

Inherent–inborn, hereditary.

Age

For most illnesses and injuries, there is more variation in disease occurrence by age than for any other variable. The study of age is thus very useful to epidemiologists. Such usefulness is largely a consequence of the association between a person's age and (1) the potential for exposure to a source of infection; (2) one's level of immunity or resistance; and (3) one's physiological activity at the tissue level, which influences the manifestation of a disease or injury. Furthermore, the efficiency of our immune system begins to decline after age twenty.

The study of mumps and measles illustrates how age influences the occurrence of infectious disease in children, who are often infected due to their lack of immunity and high risk of exposure. Table 7.1 shows the age distribution of reported mumps and the estimated incidence rates for the United States from 1985 to 1987. Most mumps cases (55.2 percent) occurred in school-age children 5 to 14 years of age, although reported mumps cases during the same time showed over an eightfold increase for 15–19 year olds. For the first time since mumps became a reportable disease, the reported peak incidence rate shifted, for two consecutive years, away from 5–9 year-old youth, which is the age group normally associated with the highest risk. The increased occurrence of mumps in susceptible adolescents and young adults has been displayed in several recent outbreaks on college campuses and in some occupational settings, primarily among those who failed to be vaccinated. Despite this age shift in the epidemiological pattern of mumps, the overall incidence of mumps in persons 10–14 and over 15 years of age is still lower than in the prevaccine and early post-vaccine licensure periods (Centers for Disease Control 1989). Thus the adoption and enforcement of universal comprehensive vaccine requirements for school attendance are most likely to substantially reduce the incidence of mumps (Table 7.2).

TABLE 7.1 Age Distribution of Reported Mumps Patients and Estimated Incidence Rates—United States, 1985–1987

Age Group (Yrs)	1985			1986			1987			Incidence Rate Change 1985–1987 (%)
	No.	(%)	Rate*	No.	(%)	Rate*	No.	(%)	Rate*	
<1	29	(1.1)	0.9	142	(2.0)	4.2	75	(0.6)	2.2	(+144.4)
1–4	339	(13.1)	2.7	569	(8.0)	4.3	729	(5.9)	5.2	(+92.6)
5–9	837	(32.5)	5.7	1768	(24.7)	11.1	2196	(17.9)	13.0	(+128.1)
10–14	649	(25.2)	4.4	2625	(36.7)	17.3	4567	(37.3)	29.0	(+559.1)
15–19	405	(15.7)	2.4	1535	(21.5)	9.0	3455	(28.2)	19.6	(+716.7)
>20	320	(12.4)	0.2	507	(7.1)	0.3	1235	(10.1)	0.8	(+300.0)
Total (known age)	2579	(100.0)	—	7146	(100.0)	—	12,257	(100.0)	—	—
Unknown age	403	—	—	644	—	—	591	—	—	—
Total	2982	—	1.1	7790	—	3.0	12,848	—	5.2	(372.7)

Source: Data from Centers for Disease Control. 1989. Mumps—United States, 1985–1988. *Morbidity and Mortality Weekly Report* 38(7):101–105.

*Rates are expressed as cases/100,000 population (projected census data) extrapolated from the age distribution of cases with known age to total cases. Not adjusted for states not reporting mumps: 1985 and 1986—Mississippi, New Mexico, Oklahoma, Oregon; 1987—Mississippi, New Mexico, Oklahoma (part-year), Oregon.

TABLE 7.2 Reported Mumps Incidence Among States, by School Immunization Laws—United States, 1985–1989

Mumps School Law Status	1985		1986		1987		1988*	
	No. States	Rate[†]	No. States	Rate[†]	No. States	Rate[†]	No. States[‡]	Rate[†]
No law	16	1.6	15	10.0	14	11.5	15	3.2
Partial law	17	1.5	17	2.0	18	6.2	18	1.9
K–12 law	14[§]	0.7	15[§]	0.7	15[§]	1.1	15[§]	1.4

Source: Data from Centers for Disease Control, 1989. Mumps—United States, 1985–1988. *Morbidity and Mortality Weekly Report* 38(7):101–105.

**1988 data represent provisional totals reported through the 52nd week.

[†]Rates are expressed as cases/100,000 population. Not adjusted for states not reporting mumps: 1985 and 1986—Mississippi, New Mexico, Oklahoma, Oregon; 1987—Mississippi, New Mexico, Oklahoma (part-year), Oregon; 1988—Mississippi, New Mexico, Oregon.

[‡]Represent classifications at the beginning of the year; during 1988, comprehensive K–12 mumps immunization requirements became effective in Wisconsin, which formerly had a K–4 requirement, and in Illinois and Tennessee, which formerly had no school immunization requirements.

[§]Includes District of Columbia.

Measles is another disease that is greatly influenced by age. During the late 1960s and early 1970s, the frequency of reported cases of measles fell dramatically in all age groups, with children less than ten years of age showing the greatest decline, while older children displayed a lesser decrease. As a consequence, the proportion of total cases occurring in different age groups displayed a change. Thus, from 1984 to 1988, 58 percent of reported cases were found in children greater than ten years of age, compared with 10 percent during the period from 1960 to 1964 (Centers for Disease Control 1989).

In 1978, a measles elimination program was initiated by the Department of Health, Education and Welfare. The goal was to eliminate indigenous measles from the United States by 1982. As a result of this program, which was aimed at the immunization of children, increased surveillance activities, and a more aggressive approach to controlling outbreaks, the number of reported cases decreased from 26,871 in 1978 to an all time low of 1,497 in 1983. By the end of 1989, however, more than 17,000 cases were reported (Centers for Disease Control 1989).

Two major types of measles outbreaks have occurred in recent years in the United States. These have involved (1) unvaccinated preschool-age children, including those younger than the recommended age of fifteen months for being vaccinated and (2) vaccinated school-age children (Markowitz et al. 1989). Additionally, in 1989 and 1990, a substantial number of cases occurred among students and personnel on college campuses. Most of the cases associated with college outbreaks were likely to have been vaccinated, although documentation was often lacking. Theoretically, vaccine failures may have occurred because an adequate response to vaccination never developed, or because an adequate response was initally developed but immunity was lost over time. Overall, the vast majority of people who are vaccinated appear to have long-term immunity (probably life-long immunity). Further studies are recommended to determine the duration of vaccine-induced immunity.

In the realm of degenerative diseases, such as type-two, non-insulin dependent diabetes, cardiovascular disease, arthritis, cancer, and Alzheimer's disease, incidence and prevalence as well as mortality rates increase proportionately with age. Once again, however, meaningful comparisons of disease occurrence in different populations can only be accomplished after statistically adjusting for differences in age distributions. Also, while it may be tempting to attribute these diseases to the aging process by itself, it should be noted that with increasing age the body has been accumulating exposure to a variety of harmful environmental influences over the years. Furthermore, as in the case of atherosclerosis and its concomitant consequences, epidemiological studies have shown that a person's habits and life-styles may significantly retard or enhance the disease process (Figure 7.3). As we discussed in Chapter 5, environmental factors play a significant role in many diseases, and this can be evidenced by the fact that incidence rates for corresponding age groups differ significantly between populations living in different environmental and cultural circumstances.

FIGURE 7.3

Danger of Heart Attack by Risk Factors Present.

Source: Framingham Heart Study, Section 37: The Probability of Developing Certain CV Diseases in Eight Years at Specified Values of Some Characteristics (Aug. 1987).

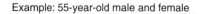

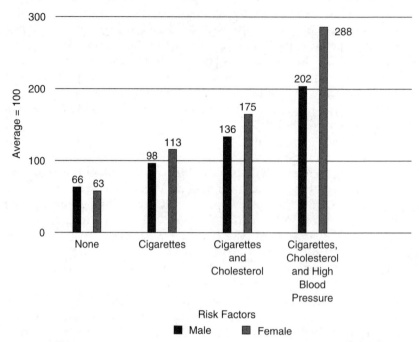

Example: 55-year-old male and female

This chart shows how a combination of three major risk factors can increase the likelihood of heart attack. For purposes of illustration, this chart uses an abnormal blood pressure level of 150 systolic and a cholesterol level of 260 in a 55-year-old male and female.

Sex

In general, males experience higher mortality rates for a wide variety of diseases than females, when rates are adjusted for age differences in the population. This becomes most evident when we examine the data obtained in Table 7.3, which compares the rates for the fifteen leading causes of death in the United States.

Mortality rates for each of the leading causes of death are higher in every instance for males, with the largest differences being the most notable for HIV infection, suicide, and homicide. Also, life expectancy at birth in 1988 for females was 78.3, as compared with 71.5 for males (U.S. Department of Health and Human Services 1990). Furthermore, it has been observed that higher male mortality is not peculiar to the United States but is common throughout the world. Usually, the differences in the death rate between the sexes are greatest in those countries where life expectancy is highest, and the differences tend to widen as a country's mortality rate declines. Evidence that greater female longevity is conditioned, in part, by the environment can be seen in newly developing countries. The poorer the overall living and health conditions are in a

TABLE 7.3 Ratio of Age-Adjusted Death Rates for the Fifteen Leading
Causes of Death by Sex and Race: United States, 1990

		Ratio of–	
Rank Order	Cause of Death, Race, and Sex (Ninth Revision, International Classification of Diseases, 1975)	Male to Female	Black to White
. . .	All causes	1.74	1.60
1	Diseases of heart	1.90	1.45
2	Malignant neoplasms, including neoplasms of lymphatic and hematopoietic tissues	1.48	1.38
3	Cerebrovascular diseases	1.18	1.90
4	Accidents and adverse effects	2.66	1.25
. . .	Motor vehicle accidents	2.46	0.99
. . .	All other accidents and adverse effects	3.01	1.61
5	Chronic obstructive pulmonary diseases and allied conditions	1.85	0.84
6	Pneumonia and influenza	1.68	1.48
7	Diabetes mellitus	1.11	2.38
8	Suicide	4.22	0.57
9	Chronic liver disease and cirrhosis	2.30	1.71
10	Human immunodeficiency virus infection	8.43	3.21
11	Homicide and legal intervention	3.88	6.69
12	Nephritis, nephrotic syndrome, and nephrosis	1.50	3.00
13	Septicemia	1.40	2.71
14	Atherosclerosis	1.33	1.15
15	Certain conditions originating in the perinatal period	1.25	3.10

Source: From U.S. Department of Health and Human Services 1993. *Monthly Vital Statistics Report* 41 (January 7):7(5).

country, as reflected by higher death rates and lower life expectancy, the smaller is the excess of female over male life expectancy.

Females, however, have significantly higher morbidity rates for most illnesses, with certain exceptions such as coronary heart disease (CHD), peptic ulcer, lung cancer and cirrhosis of the liver. Depression is also reported to be about two times greater among females, and women generally are more likely to attempt suicide than are men. It is important to note, though, that men are more apt to succeed in killing themselves than are women.

Many of these sex differences may be partly accounted for by variations in life-styles, risk-taking behavior, occupations, environment, and the acceptance of preventive medicine. However, the exact relative roles of endogenous (biological) and exogenous (environmental) factors have not yet been clearly delineated by epidemiological research.

Race and Ethnic Group

It is evident that some racial or ethnic differences in disease risk are genetically determined. For example, there is a higher rate of sickle-cell anemia in African Americans and a higher rate of cystic fibrosis in whites. However, other racial and ethnic differences observed between groups of different origins—such as infant mortality, low birth weight, AIDS, birth defects, and life expectancy—may be due more to social, economic, environmental or cultural factors rather than to biological considerations. Infant mortality rates in the United States due to birth defects are highest among Native Americans (2.9 deaths/1,000 live births) followed by Asians and Hispanics (2.6), African Americans (2.5), and whites (2.3). Overall, Asians have somewhat lower infant mortality rates (IMRs) than whites, but the rates vary from 6.0/1,000 among Japanese mothers to 9.0 among "other Asian" mothers. Hispanic mothers display an even wider variation, from 7.8 among Cubans to 12.9 among Puerto Ricans. African Americans have an IMR twice that for whites, and the rate for Native Americans is nearly 60 percent greater than that for whites. In addition, surveillance systems report that most of the HIV infections and AIDS cases among children and females of childbearing age occur among black and Hispanic populations (Centers for Disease Control 1990).

Clearly, the identification of risk factors, improved documentation of mortality differences, and effective health programs are essential if public health efforts are to succeed in reducing the burden of death, disease, and injury among these groups.

Socioeconomic Status

Socioeconomic status (SES) involves many complex interrelated variables, such as level of education obtained, income, prestige (or social standing), wealth, power, area of residence, occupation, and life-style. Information on level of education, income, occupation, and area of residence is available from a variety of sources, including the U.S. Census and special surveys. Due to practical considerations, the single attribute that is most often used in SES epidemiological studies is occupation. Great Britain, for example, has commonly delineated SES into five broad categories based on occupational or social classes: professional, intermediate, skilled, partially skilled, and unskilled occupations. In this regard, many studies show that both infant mortality and the mortality of adult males display an inverse relationship to social class.

In the United States, the poor health of minority groups is probably due largely to the disproportionate number of minorities living under conditions of poverty, with its associated problems of poor housing, poor nutrition, lack of accessibility to health services, lower environmental quality, and the general lack of knowledge concerning health conditions. For example, a recent study indicated that cholesterol screening and awareness in relationship to cardiovascular disease were significantly less among adults with low educational levels (Centers for Disease Control 1990). Similar results were obtained from analyzing data in relation to screening for mammograms (American Cancer Society 1989; Centers for Disease Control 1989). Hopefully, programs that promote the increased use of mammograms and cholesterol screening and that are targeted at lower SES segments of the population, where cancer and cardiovascular risks are often higher, should result in more positive data in the future.

Marital Status

Marital status is another variable that is routinely collected and recorded in census records, death certificates, and special surveys. According to Fox (1970), age-adjusted mortality rates for many causes of disease, for both sexes and for each sex, are generally lower for "married persons and, within each sex, higher for widowed and divorced persons." However, the lower mortality rates may reflect the better care and the more favorable environment generally experienced by married individuals as well as the observation that many individuals do not marry because of poor physical or mental health. Also, some individuals who seek risks rather than avoiding them may be less likely to marry.

Religion

Religion as a factor in disease occurrence is a very difficult variable to study, since it is compounded by different life-styles and by other personal attributes such as age, race, sex, and occupation. Mormons, for example, typify a certain way of living in regard to drinking, smoking, alcohol usage, and fitness patterns. Numerous studies have linked excessive drinking, smoking, alcohol usage, and lack of exercise to an increased risk of illness and death. This does not, however, mean that becoming a Mormon will lower one's risk of illness and death. As this example shows, one needs to use caution in interpreting data linked solely to religion as a variable in disease and illness occurrence.

Occupation

In 1987, the National Institute for Occupational Safety and Health (NIOSH) initiated the Sentinel Event Notification System for Occupation Risks (SENSOR) to improve the reporting and surveillance of work-related health conditions, such as asthma (Centers for Disease Control 1990). Asthma caused by occupational exposures has been recognized for several centuries, but the incidence and prevalence of work-induced asthma still remain unclear. Since the SENSOR program was initiated, over two hundred agents have been associated with workplace asthma. These include microbial products (such as bacillus subtillis enzymes in the detergent industry), animal proteins (such as urine protein/dander from laboratory mammals), plant products (such as wheat flour), and certain industrial chemicals. Early experience with the SENSOR program indicates that it can be a valuable tool in identifying workplaces that may contain hazardous products or chemicals that place workers at greater risk for developing occupational asthma.

Occupation as a variable in disease occurrence is another example of a factor that requires caution in interpretation, since age, sex, life-style, and other variables interact with occupation to affect the risk of disease occurrence. Obviously, certain occupations, such as mining, agriculture, and professional football, present a greater risk and exposure to accidents, injury, and death.

Life-style

Today's leading causes of death could be altered significantly by life-style changes that are designed to prevent disease and promote health. In fact, seven of the ten leading causes of death could be substantially reduced if persons at risk improved just five habits: diet, smoking, lack of exercise, alcohol abuse, and the use of antihypertensive medication (U.S. Department of Health and Human Services 1990).

Smoking, for example, is a prominent contributor to many of the ten leading causes of death: heart disease, cancer, accidents, stroke, influenza, and pneumonia. Excessive alcohol use is also involved in cancer, accidents, homicide, suicide, and cirrhosis of the liver, while improper diet is implicated in heart disease, cancer, stroke, and diabetes.

Much of our knowledge concerning behavior and health is based on epidemiological studies. Table 7.4 provides a summary list of the prominent controllable risk factors that have been identified from a variety of epidemiological studies involving health and behavior. Although such studies have established a strong cause-and-effect relationship between certain variables, many of the underlying mechanisms that explain the relationships are not yet clearly understood.

Extensive epidemiological studies have identified several factors that increase the risk of heart disease and stroke. These risk factors can be classified into two categories; major and contributing factors. *Major* risk factors are those that research has shown to be definitely associated with a significant increase in the risk of cardiovascular disease for population groups or cohorts. These include such factors as inherited traits, male sex, and increasing age. Other major factors that may be modified by altering one's life-style are cigarette smoking, high blood pressure, and elevated blood cholesterol.

Contributing risk factors include those that are associated with an increased risk of cardiovascular disease. Unfortunately, their significance and prevalence have not yet been precisely determined by vigorously controlled epidemiological investigations. Such contributing factors include diabetes, obesity, physical inactivity, and stress.

With respect to sedentary living, Powell and his colleagues (1987) reported that "sedentary groups were approximately twice as likely to die from CHD as active groups." This finding is comparable to the increased risk seen for smokers, hypertensives, and hypocholesterolemics when compared to individuals of low risk. Thus, these findings suggest that low activity levels may be as important in disease prevention as other well-known life-style indicators (Paffenbarger et al. 1986; Blair, 1989). It should be pointed out, however, that the attention given to physical activity by epidemiologists has not been as thoroughly explored as other personal

TABLE 7.4 Prominent Controllable Risk Factors in Causes of Death

Cause of Death	Risk Factors
Heart disease	Smoking, high blood pressure, elevated serum cholesterol, diabetes, obesity, lack of exercise, type A behavior (aggressive behavior patterns)
Cancers	Smoking, alcohol, solar radiation, ionizing radiation, worksite hazards, environmental pollution, medications, infectious agents, diet
Stroke	High blood pressure, cardiac function
Other than motor vehicle/accidents	Alcohol, smoking (fires), product design, home hazards, handgun availability
Influenza/pneumonia	Vaccination status, smoking
Motor vehicle/accidents	Alcohol, no safety restraints, speed, automobile design, roadway design
Diabetes	Obesity (for adult-onset)
Cirrhosis of liver	Alcohol
Suicide	Handgun availability, alcohol or drug misuse, (stress)
Homicide	Handgun availability, alcohol misuse, (stress)

Source: Modified from McGinnis, J. M. 1982. Targeting progress in health. *Public Health Reports* 97(4):298.

habits, and thus some researchers have designated sedentary living as a secondary or minor risk factor.

Karvonen (1982) observed that Finnish lumberjacks have high death rates from CHD in spite of extremely high levels of physical activity, which might lead one to conclude that physical activity would appear to have a minimal protective role. On the other hand, astute epidemiologists might argue that CHD is a multifactorial disease and thus it is unreasonable to expect that the absence of any single risk factor can provide a high degree of protection. Conversely, one may argue that high rates of a single risk factor in a population group do not necessarily ensure that the population will exhibit a high rate of CHD. For example, hypertension is prevalent in Japan, but the Japanese have low rates of CHD. Thus, in order to elevate the independent effect of a risk factor, it is necessary to observe its effect or relationship to disease within strata of another risk factor or factors.

Table 7.5 shows death rates across physical fitness levels for healthy, high risk men and women by several variables. It should be observed that the death rate declines sharply across physical fitness levels in the high risk patients. As noted by Blair (1989), "the overall rates in these high risk strata are considerably higher than for patients in low risk strata but within high risk groups, higher levels of fitness appear to provide an

TABLE 7.5 All-Cause, Age-Adjusted Death Rates Across Low, Moderate, and High Physical Fitness Levels: High Risk, Healthy Men and Women, Aerobics Center Longitudinal Study, 1970–1985

Risk Factor	Death Rates/10,000 Person-Years Physical Fitness Levels		
Men	Low	Moderate	High
Cholesterol > 260 mg/dl	95	54	27
Systolic BP > 140 mmHg	54	29	24
Current smoker	80	47	41
Women*			
Cholesterol > 260 mg/dl	83	5	25
Systolic BP > 140 mmHg	347	19	0
Current smoker	57	23	22

Source: From Blair, S., et al. 1989. Physical fitness and all-cause mortality: A prospective study of healthy men and women. *Journal of the American Medical Association* 262(17):2395-2401.

*Death rates in women are more unstable and less consistent than in men due to the small number of deaths (43) in women.

important benefit." The authors conclude that the evidence with respect to "sedentary habits and health is strong, consistent, graded, temporarily correct, specific, repeatable, independent, persistent, and biologically plausible." Accordingly, physical inactivity should perhaps be classified as one of the major risk factors for early death, which would hopefully stimulate further research by epidemiologists.

Summary

A convenient approach to describe the occurrence and distribution of disease and injury within populations is in terms of person, place, and time. These specific characteristics provide clues that might explain differing exposure to the etiological or causative agents of a disease and the varying susceptibility of population subgroups to a disease when exposure occurs. While one particular trait or characteristic of a person, such as age or sex, may predispose that individual to have an increased risk, usually several characteristics of person, place, or time interact in the development of a specific pattern of disease within a population group. Hence, it is important for epidemiologists to determine the risk of contracting a disease or injury and its association with specific characteristics of exposure and susceptibility. This information aids in the generation of hypotheses regarding the source, agent, transmission, and spread of the disease, which can then be formulated and tested through scientific methods.

Discussion Questions

1. Discuss the major factors related to time and how they may influence disease occurrence.
2. Describe how place is related to disease occurrence in populations.
3. What host attributes are related to disease occurrence?
4. Describe the major risk factors involved in coronary heart disease and how they may be modified by the host.
5. What are the major characteristics associated with point epidemics?
6. When is a true association with place suggested?
7. Describe how the epidemiology of measles has changed during the past decade.

References

American Cancer Society. 1989. Survey of awareness and use of mammograms. Princeton, NJ: The Gallup Organization.

Blair, S., H. Kohl, R. Paffenbarger, D. Clark, K. Cooper, and L. Gibbons. 1989. Physical fitness and all-cause mortality: A prospective study of healthy men and women. *Journal of the American Medical Association* 262(17):2395–2401.

Centers for Disease Control. 1990. Ectopic pregnancy—United States. *Morbidity and Mortality Weekly Report* 39(24):401–2404.

———. 1990. Factors related to cholesterol screening and cholesterol level awareness—United States, 1989. *Morbidity and Mortality Weekly Report* 39(17):634–637.

———. 1988. Human plague—United States. *Morbidity and Mortality Weekly Report* 37(42):652–656.

———. 1989. Mumps—United States; 1985–1988. *Morbidity and Mortality Weekly Report* 38(7):101–105.

———. 1990. Occupational disease surveillance: Occupational asthma. *Morbidity and Mortality Weekly Report* 39(7):119–123.

———. 1990. Reports on selected racial/ethnic groups: Special focus: Maternal and child health. *Morbidity and Mortality Weekly Report* 39(5):355.

———. 1989. Summary of notifiable diseases—United States. *Morbidity and Mortality Weekly Report* 38(54) 916–945.

———. 1989. Trends in screening mammograms for women 50 years of age and older—Behavioral risk factor surveillance system, 1987. *Morbidity and Mortality Weekly Report* 38(9):137–140.

———. 1989. Update salmonella enteritidis infections and grade A shell eggs—United States. *Morbidity and Mortality Weekly Report* 38(51):877–879.

Chow, J. 1990. The association between chlamydia trachomatis and ectopic pregnancy: A matched pair case-control study. *Journal of the American Medical Association* 263:3164–3167.

Duncan, D. 1988. *Epidemiology—Basis for disease prevention and health promotion.* New York: Macmillan.

Fox, J. et al. 1970. *Epidemiology: Man and disease.* New York: Macmillan.

Karvonen, M. 1982. Physical activity in work and leisure time in relation to cardiovascular disease. *Annals of Clinical Research* 14:118–123 (Suppl. 34).

Markowitz, L., et al. 1989. Patterns of transmission in measles—Outbreaks in the United States, 1985–86. *New England Journal of Medicine* 320:75–81.

Mausner, J., and S. Kramer. 1985. *Epidemiology: An introductory text.* Philadelphia: W. B. Saunders.

Norton, C. 1986. *Microbiology.* Menlo Park, CA: Addison-Wesley.

Office of Disease Prevention and Health Promotion. 1990. *Healthy People 2000.* DHHS Publication, No. CPHS, 90–50212. Washington, D.C.: Government Printing Office.

Paffenbarger, R., R. Hyde, A. Wing, and C. Hsieh. 1986. Physical activity, all-cause mortality, and longevity of college alumni. *New England Journal of Medicine* 314(10):605–613.

Powell, K., P. Thompson, C. Caspersen, and J. Kendrick. 1987. Physical activity and the incidence of coronary heart disease. *Annual Review of Public Health* 8:253–287.

U.S. Department of Health and Human Services. 1990. *Monthly Vital Statistics Report,* 39(7):1–48.

CHAPTER 8

Analytical Epidemiology

Introduction

Epidemiology has been defined in Chapter 1 as the study of the distribution and determinants of health-related states or events in specified populations. The study of *distribution* is largely achieved through the observational methods of epidemiology, whereas the study of *causes* is pursued through analytical and experimental methods. For the most part, the methods outlined in this chapter apply to research on morbidity and mortality problems where causes, incidence, or prevalence are usually unknown. Analytical methods can be applied to all kinds of illness, including disease, injury, mental illness, and addiction, and to physiological characteristics such as breathing capacity and blood pressure. Because most illnesses of unknown origin are noninfectious, most analytical applications focus on the major illnesses of this kind, such as heart disease and cancer. But the emergence from time to time of new infectious diseases, such as Lyme disease and AIDS, has spurred researchers to use methods of analytical epidemiology to investigate those diseases as well.

The basic research question for all epidemiological studies of cause is: Does exposure to the agent cause disease? All research begins with carefully defined and logical research questions or propositions, which are usually derived from a sound theoretical base. If the propositions are precise, logical, theoretically sound, and testable they are called **hypotheses**. An example of a hypothesis would be as follows: to test the hypothesis that U.S. white males aged thirty-five to fifty-nine with ischemic heart disease are *exposed* to cigarettes at higher rates (twenty or more cigarettes per day for ten years), than U.S. white males without the disease. To answer research questions, the investigator sets specific tasks or objectives, for example: to measure the **rate of exposure** to benzene during an eight-hour workday of workers in a paint factory.

Because epidemiology deals mainly with human populations it cannot conduct true experimental studies, except for some types of clinical trials. There have been deplorable instances of human experimentation among populations of hospitals, prisons, concentration camps, and other

Hypothesis–a supposition arrived at from observation or reflection put forth to account for known facts, which may serve as a starting point for further investigation by which it may be proved or disproved and the true theory arrived at (*Oxford English Dictionary*).

Rate of exposure–the intensity or concentration of an agent in the environment and the duration of time during which a person is exposed to it. For example: 50 parts per million per cubic meter of air for 15 minutes.

institutions, but these are rare exceptions. Circumstances sometimes permit the study of what is, for epidemiologists, an unplanned "experiment." The atomic bombings of Japan; severe famines; disasters such as the release of toxic gases at Bhopal in India and radiation at Chernobyl, Russia; and comparisons of migrating and nonmigrating populations are all opportunities for epidemiological studies. Quasi-experiments in populations are possible in limited ways. For example, new vaccines and therapeutic drugs can be tested in experimental trials. Most epidemiological research uses methods that observe **exposures** to agents and illness effects without manipulating the population under study. These are called analytical methods and we will deal with them first. For more detailed treatments of analytical methods, reference should be made to more advanced general texts (Lilienfeld and Lilienfeld and Stolley 1994; Mausner and Kramer 1985), or specialized texts (Kelsey, Thompson, and Evans 1986; Schlesselman 1982).

Exposure–the presence in the environment of the agent or agents associated with or causing illness in populations. An individual is exposed when in the presence of an agent.

Analytical Methods

The main objective of epidemiological research is to discover the cause and distribution of illness in populations. All the analytical methods help epidemiologists pursue this objective by observing the experience of a particular population over time. Through the various methods, epidemiologists are able to observe the exposure of the population to agents suspected of causing an illness and then determine the occurrence or rate of illness. The differences between the methods are important more for choice of application to different problems and for logistical reasons, rather than for theoretical considerations.

Case Series

The simplest method is a case series, which is prompted by an observation of what appears to be an unusual number of cases of an illness in a population at a particular time and place. This may take the form of a **geographical cluster** of cases in a community or a group of cases in one situation, such as a factory or a school. One of the key questions in determining whether or not the observed cases are unusual is: What is the incidence rate? To answer this question, the epidemiologist needs to be knowledgeable in regard to the normal occurrence of this particular disease. For instance, is this disease expressing itself in the population in excess of what is normally expected? This requires knowing the population at risk (the denominator for the rate), the number of cases of illness or death (the numerator), and the normal distribution of this disease in the population under study. The true population at risk may be difficult to determine, especially if the case series has appeared in a general community. It is usually easier to establish the true population at risk if the cases are confined to an institution such as a school or factory. If the illness in question is a rare disease, such as mesothelioma, which is almost always caused by exposure to certain asbestos fibers, or angiosarcoma of the liver, which is invariably caused by industrial exposure

Geographical cluster–an aggregation of cases of a disease, or other health-related condition, which are closely grouped in a geographical area such as a neighborhood or city district, school, shopping center, or industrial area.

to vinyl chloride gas, a series of cases by itself is strongly suggestive of cause. An investigation of the intensity and duration of the exposure of the cases to the suspected agents is carried out. This may provide sufficient evidence for concluding the study, or it may indicate the need for more work.

Cohort Studies

A cohort is a particular population, and in epidemiology this is the study population in which agents and illness are to be observed. The cohort study design is sometimes called "longitudinal," "prospective," and "incidence," but cohort is the name most widely used. The term *cohort* has been restricted by some epidemiologists to a group of people of similar age, but it is more often used to refer to the entire available study population. In an epidemiological cohort study, the population is observed over time, and exposure to agents and outcomes of illness are recorded. This is analogous to an experimental design in which the agents are identified, the population and its exposure to the agents are followed over time, and illness outcomes are observed among persons exposed and not exposed. The incidence rates in exposed, and in non-exposed groups of the population can then be calculated and compared.

The incidence rate in the population actually exposed to an agent is called the **absolute risk**. For example, the absolute risk for nasal cancer in a population of furniture workers actually exposed to hardwood dust for 20 years might be 120 per 1,000 workers. The ratio of the incidence rate in the population exposed to an agent, to the incidence rate in the population not exposed to it, is called the **relative risk** (Table 8.1).

In cohort studies, the time period of observation in the study population can begin at some point in the past and then be followed to the present. This is called a *historical* or *retrospective* cohort study. Or, the cohort is followed from the present time into some point in the future—a *prospective* cohort study (Example 8.1). In theory, a prospective cohort study is preferred because the agents and population exposures can be observed as they happen. This design is often impractical, however, because the numbers of cases of illness that occur in a reasonable time period may be too small to draw valid conclusions.

The cost of cohort studies is usually comparatively high, in that they involve following large numbers of people for a sufficient time for illness to occur. In diseases with long latency periods, the time may have to be ten or more years. In historical cohort studies, there is usually the advantage of being able to identify a large number of cases of the illness under study beforehand, so that estimated costs are known before an expensive study is undertaken. Epidemiologists that have investigated disasters, such as the atomic bombings of Japan, can first conduct a historical cohort study and then continue with a prospective study, if resources permit and the problem justifies it. Good examples of cohort studies are those associated with entire communities, such as Framingham, Massachusetts, and Tecumseh, Michigan, where exposures to agents associated with a variety of diseases have been investigated for more than thirty years (Epstein et al. 1970).

Absolute risk–the incidence rate of a particular illness or cause of death in a population exposed to an agent or a risk factor.

Relative risk–the ratio comparing the incidence rate of a particular illness or cause of death in the group of a population exposed to an agent or a risk factor, to the incidence rate in the group of the population not exposed to it. Relative risk is a measure of the effect, or relative weight, of an agent or a risk factor associated with a particular illness or cause of death.

TABLE 8.1 Calculating Relative and Attributable Risk

$$\text{Relative risk} = \frac{\text{Incidence rate among exposed}}{\text{Incidence rate among non-exposed}}$$

Using the example of furniture workers, where the rate among exposed was 120 per 1,000 workers, and assuming the rate among non-exposed was 5 per 1,000 workers, the relative risk for nasal cancer would be:

$$\text{Relative risk} = \frac{120 \text{ per } 1,000 \text{ workers}}{5 \text{ per } 1,000 \text{ workers}} = 24.0$$

The number or proportion of cases of illness or cause of death attributable to an agent is called the *attributable risk*. Attributable risk can be calculated either for the exposed population or for the total population, multiplied by 100 to be expressed as a percentage.

$$\text{Attributable risk in exposed population} = \frac{\begin{array}{c}\text{Incidence rate in exposed population} - \\ \text{Incidence rate in non-exposed population}\end{array}}{\text{Incidence rate in exposed population}} \times 100$$

$$\text{Attributable risk in total population} = \frac{\begin{array}{c}\text{Incidence rate in exposed population} - \\ \text{Incidence rate in non-exposed population}\end{array}}{\begin{array}{c}\text{Incidence rate in exposed population} + \\ \text{Incidence rate in non-exposed population}\end{array}} \times 100$$

In the example of furniture workers, the attributable risk in the exposed population would be:

$$\frac{120 - 5}{120} \times 100 = 96\%$$

And in the total population:
$$\frac{120 - 5}{120 + 5} \times 100 = 92\%$$

Case-Control Studies

Risk factor–an aspect of personal behavior or life-style, an environmental exposure, or an inborn or inherited characteristic that is associated with an increased occurrence of disease or other health-related event or condition. A risk factor is not necessarily a causal factor.

With this design, the illness outcome is already known in a group of cases. The epidemiologist then obtains histories of exposure to suspected agents in the cases and compares these with histories of exposure in a group of controls without illness. The number of controls is usually the same as the number of cases, but it may be larger. In one variation of this design, the control participants are individually matched to cases by sex, age, and other criteria to form matched pairs. Or, two or more controls may be matched to a single case. These techniques are used to improve statistical power, because all case-control studies are *samples* of the study population experience over time. This is in contrast to the cohort study, which observes the *total* study population. The results of a case-control study are expressed as the chance, or odds, of the cases' illness being associated with exposure to the suspected agent, or **risk factor**. The **odds**

To assess levels of continual physical exertion in relation to the risk of fatal heart attack, a prospective cohort study was conducted among 6,351 long-shoremen in the San Francisco Bay area (Paffenbarger and Hale 1975).

The men, aged 35–74 years, were followed for 22 years (1951 to 1972), or to death, or to the age of 75. Their longshoring experience was computed in terms of work years according to categories of high, medium, and low caloric output. The age-adjusted coronary death rates for the high activity category was 26.9 per 10,000 work years, and the medium and low categories had rates of 46.3 and 49.0. The death rates for sudden fatal heart attack among the high activity workers was 5.6, among the moderate activity workers it was 19.9, and among the light activity workers it was 15.7. The study concluded that repeated bursts of high energy output had a protective effect against coronary mortality.

Odds ratio–a ratio measure of the association between factors, used in epidemiology to indicate the probability of exposure to a suspected agent or risk factor. It is an estimate of the relative risk. An odds ratio of 1.0 indicates that exposure was the same in the groups being compared, for example, cases and controls. An odds ratio of 5.0 indicates that exposure in cases was five times that of controls, and an odds ratio of 0.5 that exposure in controls was twice that of cases.

Validity–the degree to which a measurement actually measures or detects what it is supposed to measure.

ratio is an estimate of the *relative risk* and is a good indicator of the magnitude of the effect of the agent (see terminology).

A case-control design is generally much less expensive than a cohort study, because it limits exposure assessment to the cases of an illness and to a sample of the study population that generated the cases. If the controls are randomly sampled from the total study population, the design is called a *cohort-based case-control study*. With this particular design, bias and other statistical concerns can be well-controlled, so that the **validity** of results will be no less than those obtained from a cohort study. On the other hand, if the controls are sampled from a convenient subpopulation, such as those in a disease registry or from patients in a hospital, the validity of the results may be considerably less. These kinds of studies are called *registry- or hospital-based case-control studies*.

Case-control studies are particularly useful for studying comparatively rare and fatal diseases with long induction and latency periods, such as most cancers (Example 8.2). Thus, they are preferred over cohort studies for these situations. They are not suited, though, for studies of nonfatal illnesses where onset and end point are often uncertain.

Proportionate Mortality or Morbidity Studies

Sometimes it is not possible for epidemiologists to find control participants to compare with the cases of an illness. One alternative is to use mortality data from death certificates that come from the general population. For some diseases, such as cancer, population-based registries can provide incidence data for a proportionate morbidity study. The proportions of mortality (or morbidity) in the study group of cases are then compared with the corresponding proportions in the reference population, for

In 1980, in Malaysia, a case-control study among Malaysian Chinese investigated the association between eating salted fish in childhood and contracting cancer of the nasopharynx in adulthood (Armstrong et al. 1983). A matched-pairs design was used with 100 disease cases matched by sex and age to 100 non-disease control participants. All participants were interviewed about present and past dietary patterns, including their consumption of salted fish. The frequency of cases and controls consuming various foods was compared, and odds ratios were calculated as estimates of relative risk. The relative risk for ever having eaten salted fish in childhood was 3.0; and the relative risks for never eating, eating less than daily, and eating daily were, 1.0, 2.8, and 17.4, respectively. All results were statistically significant.

The results indicated that eating salted fish was associated 2.8 times more with disease cases than with non-disease controls, and eating it daily was associated 17.4 times more. The association was confirmed by subsequent studies in Hong Kong and in China. In addition, laboratory studies have since demonstrated that salted fish from Southeast Asia, which may be contaminated with nitrosamines that are carcinogenic in animals, can cause nasal cancers in laboratory animals.

example, the population of the United States or of Illinois. The comparison produces proportionate mortality ratios, which indicate the magnitude of the difference of illness effect between the exposed case group and the general reference population (Example 8.3).

Cross-Sectional (Prevalence) Studies

In this design the prevalence, rather than the incidence, of the illness under study is surveyed at one point or period of time. Cross-sectional studies are done once (a one-time survey) or may be repeated at intervals as a series of cross-sectional studies. If these repeated surveys observe the same study group each time, they are sometimes called *panel studies.*

Cross-sectional studies are generally the best choice for investigations of nonfatal illnesses, or of physiological or psychological responses to agents. In these illnesses, the time of initiation and recovery may be uncertain, so incidence cannot be determined, but determining prevalence at a point or period of time is a practical and valuable measure. In a cross-sectional study, the study population is defined and the prevalence of the study illness is determined in association with subpopulations exposed, and not exposed, to suspected causal agents (Example 8.4).

EXAMPLE 8.3

Dalager, Mason, and Fraumeni (1980) compared the observed number of deaths from respiratory cancer in 202 male painters exposed to zinc chromate with the number of deaths expected among the United States male population. The proportionate mortality ratios in this study indicated that an increased risk of respiratory cancer was associated with duration of employment among the painters.

EXAMPLE 8.4

A cross-sectional study was done of the relationship of respiratory symptoms to air pollution (suspended particulates and oxides of sulfur) in a random sample of 866 women, 25 years of age or older, in Buffalo, New York, during the period from 1961 to 1963 (Winkelstein and Kantos 1969). Smokers had higher rates of cough with phlegm than nonsmokers, and nonsmokers who were 45 years of age or older had higher rates of cough with phlegm in association with exposure to particulate air pollution. There was no positive association between respiratory symptoms and oxides of sulfur air pollution.

Other Analytical Issues

All analytical study designs in epidemiology are essentially observational, rather than experimental, which means that they cannot test hypotheses definitively or provide proof of causal relationships. Instead, they offer evidence of association between illness in the population and exposure to agents. The replication of studies provides reinforcing (or conflicting) evidence, but because the various research settings cannot be duplicated exactly, replication still does not provide proof. Other evidence must be brought to bear to substantiate the epidemiological evidence, such as demonstrating a physiological mechanism linking the agent to a pathological outcome, or providing evidence from laboratory studies in animals that the suspected agent can cause the disease in other species. This kind of substantiation has come about for such causal factors as cigarette smoking with heart disease and respiratory disease, sunlight and fair skin with skin cancers, and several chemical substances with a variety of occupationally related diseases.

While the general design of analytical methods in epidemiology is simple, the chances of random and systematic error are complex and of considerable concern to researchers. *Random errors* affect the precision of a study and must be minimized by using as large a study population, or sample of a study population, as possible. The probability of random error can be calculated by statistical methods (Streiner 1986). *Systematic errors*, or bias, come from errors in the selection of the study participants; from errors in the classification of the participants in respect to their reporting of exposure to agents; and in errors of confounding, when the exposed and non-exposed study groups are not comparable. Epidemiologists try to guard against systematic errors by carefully designing and executing their studies. These topics are covered in texts dealing with the statistical design and analysis of epidemiological studies (Kahn and Sempos 1989; Kelsey, Thompson, and Evans 1986; Schlesselman 1982).

Experimental Trials

In true experiments there is direct control of all factors involved. In epidemiology, this would mean having direct control over populations, agents of illness, and the environment. As we stressed earlier, it is not acceptable to carry out direct experimentation on human populations. What is acceptable, however, is a quasi-experimental design in which the investigator has direct control over the assignment of individuals to study groups. In a quasi-experimental design, there are usually two study groups. One is called the *experimental* group, which is given the drug or procedure to be tested. The other is the *control* group, which is given the drug currently in use or, if there is no established drug, a harmless substitute **(placebo)**, such as a sugar pill. After waiting an appropriate time interval, the experimental and control groups are followed up and the effect of the drug or procedure being tested is evaluated. This form of epidemiological experiment is called a *trial*. It has been most effectively applied in testing therapeutic drugs or other procedures to treat disease (therapeutic trials); in testing drugs that reduce the risk of disease, such as those that control hypertension and thereby reduce the risk of fatal vascular diseases (intervention trials); and in testing vaccines to prevent disease (preventive trials).

Placebo–a harmless substitute for the real thing, for example, a sugar pill instead of an aspirin tablet.

These three different applications of trials may all be carried out in two general ways: (1) as *clinical trials,* in which the effect of the drug or procedure is tested in individual members of the experimental and control groups, and (2) as *community trials,* in which the groups as a whole are the subject of the test. The most important distinguishing characteristic of clinical trials, as compared to cohort studies, is that the individuals in the experimental and control groups are randomly assigned to the groups. In this way, the investigator can control the comparability of the two groups, so that they are similar in all factors except the one being tested, that is, the drug or procedure. The design and execution of experimental trials is complex; for more in-depth treatment, reference can be made to Hill (1962) and Meinert (1986).

Special Studies

Some situations afford a special opportunity to epidemiologists to carry out research. One of these situations is the phenomenon of human migration. When a population of one country migrates to another, which is culturally very different, and establishes itself in the new environment, there are often changes in the frequency patterns of illness in the migrants as compared to the population left behind in the homeland. Not surprisingly, the changes are more rapid in illnesses that are primarily of environmental origin and are less rapid in those of genetic origin. The first generation of adult migrants tends to retain the illness patterns of its homeland, although being a select group that chose or was obliged to migrate, these adults are often more resistant to illness and healthier than those who remained. However, the illness patterns of the adult migrants are often markedly different from those of the population they have settled with. The children, more so than their parents, tend to adopt many of the customs of their new homeland, especially diet. Succeeding generations tend to represent more and more of the culture and environment of the new land.

Since 1950, several substantial migrations have been the subject of epidemiological research. These include Britons who migrated to Australia and New Zealand; Chinese, Japanese, Filipinos, Samoans, and Vietnamese who migrated to the United States; Poles and Scandinavians who migrated to Canada and the United States; Europeans of many countries who migrated to Israel; Tokelau Islanders who migrated to New Zealand; and others. The results of comparing populations who have migrated and their descendents with those in the old and new homelands has given important evidence of the significance of environmental factors in causing cancers of the lung, stomach, and colon; hypertension; and cardiovascular disease. As we saw in Chapter 5, Table 5.3, there are marked differences between countries in the incidence of major cancers. The first generation of migrants from a low incidence country to a high incidence one usually shows little change in incidence rates from the homeland patterns. However, where environmental factors such as diet, habits of exercise, smoking and alcohol use, and occupations are important in the etiology of certain illnesses, the descendents of migrants show a shift in incidence rates toward those of the established population. In fact, differences in rates may be insignificant by the second generation.

One of the most important epidemiological studies ever undertaken is the ongoing follow-up study of the survivors of the atomic bombings of Hiroshima and Nagasaki, Japan, in 1945. Japanese, American, and other scientists began this study shortly after the bombings. It has provided vital information about the immediate and long-term health effects of nuclear weapons on human populations, and about the particular combinations of radioactive isotopes that are generated in these explosions. [In order to extrapolate the information learned about radiation exposure in the environment and about radiation *dosage* to human cells in the study

Dose–dose can have various meanings in epidemiology, ranging from the amount of a substance or radioisotope that remains in body cells or tissues for some specified time period, to the amount of a substance taken into the body, as in a "dose of medicine."

populations to other populations, the investigators developed models of exposure, dosage, and disease process.] The disease of prime interest has been cancer, because it is the most serious end result for the long-term survivors. The process of extrapolating likely disease outcomes and the probability of disease is called *risk assessment*. This has now become an important branch of occupational and environmental epidemiology, but the theory and methods were first worked out in radiation studies.

Other special studies of significance are those based on the long-term observation of particular communities. Framingham, Massachusetts, and Tecumseh, Michigan, have already been mentioned. Alameda County, California, and Karelia County in Finland are others (Berkman and Breslow 1983). Studies of hypertension and cardiovascular disease risks have been especially noteworthy in these communities and have helped to confirm the importance of such risk factors as cigarette smoking, diets high in saturated fats, and cholesterol. Communities with distinctive dietary habits or taboos have also provided opportunities for epidemiologists to do contrasting studies with the habits representing the majority culture. For example, the Mormon and Seventh Day Adventist communities, with their restrictions on alcohol, coffee, and other food items, have been the subject of comparative study (Polednak 1989).

Summary

The basic research question in epidemiology is: Does exposure to the agent cause illness in the population? Because epidemiologists deal with human populations, they cannot undertake direct experiments and therefore use primarily observational methods. Five kinds of analytical methods are used to observe the exposure of a study population to suspected causal agents over time and determine the occurrence of illness. (1) The case-series is the study of a group of cases of illness or death and the rate and duration of exposure they experienced to suspected agents. (2) The cohort study involves the observation of an entire population over time and records the exposure to agents and outcomes of an illness. It leads to finding the incidence rates of the illness in population subgroups who were exposed and not exposed to the agents. (3) The case-control study begins with a group of cases in which the illness outcome is known. Epidemiologists then establish case histories of exposure to suspected agents and compare these with histories of exposure in a group of controls without illness. A case-control study leads to an estimate of the relative risk or magnitude of the effect of an agent in association with illness in the cases. (4) Proportionate mortality or morbidity studies compare the proportions of mortality (or morbidity) in a group of cases exposed to a suspected agent with the proportions in a general reference population. The resultant proportionate mortality (or morbidity) ratio indicates the magnitude of the difference of illness effect between the exposed case group and the general reference population. (5) Cross-sectional studies establish the prevalence of illness at one point in time in population subgroups that are exposed and not exposed to suspected causal agents.

In limited ways, epidemiologists conduct quasi-experiments called trials, in which individuals are randomly assigned to study groups. One group, called the experimental group, is given the new drug, vaccine, or procedure to be tested, while the other group, called the control group, is given the current drug, vaccine, procedure, or a placebo. After an appropriate time interval, the two groups are followed up and the effect of the test is evaluated. Epidemiological research has also been done on "unplanned experiments," as in comparisons of exposures to agents and incidence rates of illness and death among migrants and nonmigrant populations, and in the follow-up of particular populations exposed to agents in disasters, such as the atomic bombings of Japan and the chemical pollution of Bhopal, India. Certain geographical and religious communities have also been the subject of comparative studies to evaluate the relative importance of risk factors in heart disease and other noninfectious diseases.

Discussion Questions

1. In a case-control study of lung cancer, the 200 cases and 200 controls with, and without, a history of smoking over 30 cigarettes per day for 10 years were distributed as follows:

Cigarettes Per Day	Cases	Controls	Calculate the Odds Ratio
30 or more	160 (a)	80 (b)	$$\dfrac{\dfrac{a}{(a + b)}}{\dfrac{c}{(c + d)}} = \dfrac{ad}{bc} = \text{answer}$$
Less than 30	40 (c)	120 (d)	

What does the result mean? The odds ratio is an estimate of the relative risk. What is the relative risk? What does the relative risk in this example tell us about the possible magnitude of the effect of smoking for lung cancer?

2. The incidence rate of byssinosis in a group of textile workers actually exposed to cotton dusts for 8 hours per workday for 20 years was 60 per 1,000 workers, while the incidence rate in a group of textile workers not exposed was 3 per 1,000. Calculate the (a) absolute risk, (b) relative risk, (c) attributable risk in the exposed population, and (d) attributable risk in the total population.

3. What are the differences between clinical trials and community trials?

4. Compare and contrast case-control, cohort, and cross-sectional study designs.

References

Armstrong, R. W., M. J. Armstrong, M. C. Yu, and B. E. Henderson. 1983. Salted fish and inhalants as risk factors for nasopharyngeal carcinoma in Malaysian Chinese. *Cancer Research* 43:2967–2970.

Berkman, L. F., and L. Breslow. 1983. *Health and ways of living: The Alameda county study.* New York: Oxford University Press.

Dalager, N. A., T. J. Mason, and J. F. Fraumeni. 1980. Cancer mortality among workers exposed to zinc chromate paints. *Journal of Occupational Medicine* 22:25–29.

Epstein, F. H., J. A. Napier, W. D. Block, N. S. Hayner, M. P. Higgins, B. C. Johnson, J. B. Keller, H. L. Metzner, H. J. Montoyne, L. D. Ostrander, and B. M. Ullman. 1970. The Tecumseh study. *Archives of Environmental Health,* 21:402–407.

Hill, A. B. 1962. *Statistical methods in clinical and preventive medicine.* Edinburgh: Churchill Livingstone.

Kahn, H. A., and C. T. Sempos. 1989. *Statistical methods in epidemiology.* New York: Oxford University Press.

Kelsey, J. L., W. D. Thompson, and A. S. Evans. 1986. *Methods in observational epidemiology.* New York: Oxford University Press.

Lilienfeld, D. E. and P. D. Stolley. 1994. *Foundations of epidemiology,* 3rd ed. New York: Oxford University Press.

Mausner, J. S., and S. Kramer. 1985. *Epidemiology: An introductory text,* 2nd ed. Philadelphia: W. B. Saunders.

Meinert, C. L. 1986. *Clinical trials.* New York: Oxford University Press.

Paffenbarger, R. S., and W. E. Hale. 1975. Work activity and coronary heart mortality. *New England Journal of Medicine* 292:545–550.

Polednak, A. P. 1989. *Racial and ethnic differences in disease.* New York: Oxford University Press.

Schlesselman, J. J. 1982. *Case-control studies.* New York: Oxford University Press.

Streiner, N. 1986. *PDQ Statistics.* 1986. Toronto: Decker.

Winkelstein, W., and S. Kantos. 1969. Respiratory symptoms and air pollution in an urban population of northeastern United States. *Archives of Environmental Health* 18:760–767.

CHAPTER 9

Epidemiology and Sexually Transmitted Diseases

Introduction

Do Americans enjoy better health today than they did twenty or thirty years ago? In general, we would all say "of course." We know, however, that the life-styles of many individuals include a number of risk taking behaviors. Our grandparents took many necessary risks in their attempts to survive. Today, however, many life-styles are filled with unnecessary risks, especially given what we know about disease and prevention. Excess alcohol and drug consumption, for example, places many individuals at risk for exposure to organisms such as bacteria and viruses as well as to accidents, homicides, and suicides.

This chapter will focus on the risk that is posed by several sexually transmitted diseases (STDs). These include AIDS, chlamydia, **genital herpes**, **genital warts**, gonorrhea, nonspecific urethritis (NSU), pubic lice, and syphilis. The new wave of STDs, the sexual aspects of cancer risk, AIDS, and acquaintance rape are some of the significant life-style risks found in our society today.

Acquired Immunodeficiency Syndrome (AIDS)

In June 1981, the first cases of AIDS were reported in five young Los Angeles homosexual men diagnosed with **pneumocystis carinii pneumonia** and other **opportunistic infections**. Earlier, however, isolated cases had occurred in the United States and in several other areas of the world, including Haiti, Africa, and Europe during the 1970s. By mid-1990, over 130,000 cases had been reported in the United States (Benenson 1990).

On a worldwide basis, the World Health Organization (WHO) estimates that 13 million men, women and children have been infected with the human immunodeficiency virus (HIV). Each day, approximately 5,000 persons are newly infected, and by the year 2000, it is estimated that 40 million persons could be infected (Centers for Disease Control 1993).

Genital herpes–a painful infection of the genitals (herpes genitalis) caused by the herpes simplex virus. Groups of blisters develop on one or several areas. These blisters eventually rupture and become shallow ulcers or sores. Herpes genitalis is transmitted through sexual activity and through contaminated hands.

Genital warts–genital or venereal warts (condyloma acuminatum) are very common. They are caused by the papilloma virus and are usually transmitted by direct sexual contact. These painless warts appear one to two months after exposure.

Pneumocystis carinii pneumonia–this type of pneumonia is caused by a virulent protozoa. It is characterized by an abrupt or gradual onset of symptoms and a temperature of about 104°F (40°C). Rapid breathing, cough and shortness of breath are symptoms of this opportunistic infection.

Opportunistic infection–an infection in an immuno-suppressed person caused by an organism that does not usually trouble people with healthy immune systems.

Who Is at Risk?

In 1990, AIDS ranked seventh among the causes of estimated years of potential life loss before age 65 (Centers for Disease Control 1992). In 1992, AIDS ranked eighth among the leading causes of death. Of the approximately 33,590 HIV infection deaths that year, 60 percent were white males, 27 percent were African-American males, 5 percent were white females, and 8 percent were African-American females. The largest number of deaths from AIDS, for both males and females, were in the age group of 25–44 years. Although the number for deaths was the highest for white males, the age-adjusted death rates and almost all age-specific death rates were the highest for African-American males, followed by white males, African-American females, and white females. Between 1991 and 1992, the increase in the age-adjusted death rates was larger for African-American females than for African-American males and white males, with little change occurring for white females (National Center for Health Statistics 1993).

Among males in 1992, 60 percent of the cases of AIDS occurred among men who had sex with men (homosexual and bisexual), with an additional 21 percent of cases being reported by males who injected drugs. Among females (Figure 9.1), 45 percent of the cases were found in women who reported injecting drugs, and 39 percent were traced to heterosexual contact (Centers for Disease Control 1993). From 1981 through 1993, however, the proportion of persons with AIDS who reported heterosexual contact with a partner at risk for or with documented HIV infection increased from 1.9 percent to 9.0 percent (Figure 9.2). During the same time period, the proportion of cases attributed to male sexual contact decreased from 66.5 percent to 46.6 percent, while the proportion attributed to intravenous drug users (IDUs) among women and heterosexual men increased from 17.4 percent to 27.7 percent.

In 1993, most heterosexually acquired AIDS cases were associated with heterosexual contact with an IDU (42.3 percent) or with a partner with HIV infection or AIDS whose risk was not reported or known (Figure 9.3). The number of cases attributed to heterosexual contact with bisexual males, transfusion or transplant recipients, or persons with hemophilia was relatively small. Table 9.1 presents the number and percentage of persons with heterosexually acquired AIDS, by race/ethnicity and percentage increase from 1992 to 1993. The highest proportion of U.S. cases associated with heterosexual contact during 1993 occurred in the south (42 percent) and the northeast (31 percent); these areas also account for 24 percent and 53 percent, respectively, of cases reported among heterosexual intraveneous drug users (Centers for Disease Control 1994).

Quinn (1993), in addressing the issue of risk factors and HIV infection, stresses the need to "acknowledge the existence of a serious gap in our knowledge base on women and AIDS," since there appears to be a scarcity of systemic, population-based data on knowledge, attitudes,

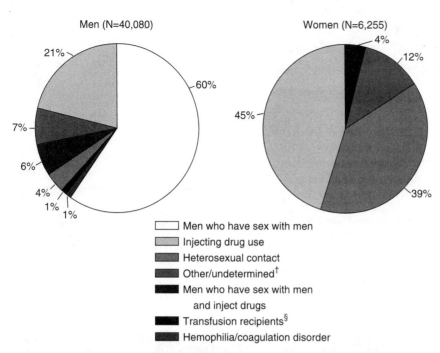

Men (N=40,080)

60%
21%
7%
6%
4%
1%
1%

Women (N=6,255)

4%
12%
45%
39%

☐ Men who have sex with men
▨ Injecting drug use
▨ Heterosexual contact
▨ Other/undetermined†
■ Men who have sex with men
    and inject drugs
■ Transfusion recipients§
▨ Hemophilia/coagulation disorder

FIGURE 9.1
Acquired Immunodeficiency Syndrome (AIDS)–Reported Adult/Adolescent Cases, by Exposure Category and Sex, United States,* 1992.

Source: Centers for Disease Control, MMWR, Summary of Notifiable Diseases, United States-1992, 41:55,1993.

*Includes Guam, Puerto Rico, the U.S. Pacific Islands, and the U.S. Virgin Islands.

†"Other" refers to persons who developed AIDS after exposure to HIV-infected blood within the health-care setting, as documented evidence of seroconversion or other laboratory studies. "Undetermined" refers to patients whose mode of exposure to HIV is unknown. This includes patients under investigation; patients who died, were lost to follow-up, or refused interview; and patients whose mode of exposure to HIV remains undetermined after investigation.

§Includes transfusion, tissue, and organ recipients from donors who were screened negative for HIV antibody at the time of donation.

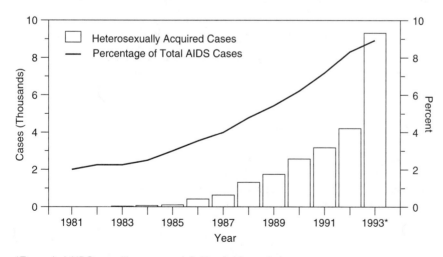

□ Heterosexually Acquired Cases
— Percentage of Total AIDS Cases

FIGURE 9.2
Number of AIDS Cases Attributed to Heterosexual HIV Transmission and Percentage of Total AIDS Cases—United States, 1981–1993.

Source: Centers for Disease Control, MMWR, 43:9,1994.

*Expanded AIDS surveillance case definition implemented.

Epidemiology and Sexually Transmitted Diseases   117

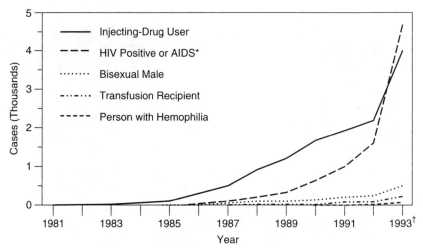

FIGURE 9.3
Number of AIDS Cases Attributed to Heterosexual HIV Transmission, by Partner's Risk Factor—United States, 1981–1993.

Source: Centers for Disease Control, MMWR, 43:9, 1994.

*Partner's risk unknown or not reported.
†Expanded AIDS surveillance case definition implemented.

TABLE 9.1 Number and Percentage of Adolescents and Adults with Heterosexually Acquired AIDS, by Race/Ethnicity and Percentage Increase—United States, 1992–1993

	Males			Females		
Race/Ethnicity	1992 No. (%)	1993 No.(%)	% Increase from 1992 to 1993	1992 No. (%)	1993 No. (%)	% Increase from 1992 to 1993
White, non-Hispanic	331 (22)	681 (21)	106	616 (24)	1510 (25)	145
Black, non-Hispanic	845 (56)	1789 (55)	112	1308 (52)	3022 (50)	131
Hispanic	325 (22)	736 (23)	126	584 (23)	1444 (24)	147
Asian/Pacific Islander	3 (<1)	16 (<1)	*	20 (<1)	52 (<1)	*
American Indian/Alaskan Native	1 (<1)	6 (<1)	*	5 (<1)	23 (<1)	*
Total†	1509 (100)	3232 (100)	114	2536 (100)	6056 (100)	139

Source: From Centers for Disease Control. 1994. Morbidity and Mortality Weekly Report 43:9.

*Estimate of percentage change is unreliable because of small numbers of cases.

†Includes eight men and eight women for whom race/ethnicity was unknown.

and behavior. Such data could serve to further our understanding of the spread of HIV disease.

According to the Centers for Disease Control and Prevention, approximately 59 percent of heterosexually transmitted cases among African-American women are the result of being the sex partner of an IDU. The cumulative incidence of AIDS cases acquired through heterosexual contact are more than eleven times higher for African-American women than for white women (Holmes, Karon, and Kaeiss 1990).

While the association between intravenous drug use and HIV infection is well-established, one should note that for female IDUs, the risk of HIV infection stems from multiple factors, such as sharing contaminated needles as well as being more likely to be poly-drug abusers. In addition, women's use of crack cocaine specifically increases their participation in unprotected sexual activity, and these women are also more likely to participate in risk behaviors such as multiple sex partners, prostitution, and the exchange of sex for drugs. Furthermore, women who are IDUs are more likely to have a primary relationship with a male IDU and are susceptible to physical abuse and rape, which may place them at greater risk (Karin 1989). It is clear that prevention efforts need to be expanded in order to implement effective HIV education strategies that can reduce the risk of HIV infections in populations participating in known risk behaviors.

In 1990, for San Francisco, Los Angeles, New York City, and Baltimore, HIV infection/AIDS was the leading cause of death among young adult men, surpassing heart disease, cancer, and homicide (Centers for Disease Control 1991). Although larger metropolitan areas report most of the AIDS cases, smaller cities and rural areas are increasingly reporting a large number of cases. Before 1986, metropolitan statistical areas with less than 500,000 population reported 10 percent of all AIDS cases, as compared to 19 percent in 1988.

Surveillance

All fifty states and the District of Columbia require health–care providers to report new cases of AIDS to their respective state health departments. HIV infection reports are useful in directing HIV-related prevention activities, such as partner notification, client counseling, and referral for appropriate medical management. HIV infection reports are also useful for guiding pediatric medical and social support programs as well as programs for infants, whose infection status may remain undetermined until they are 15 months or more in age (Centers for Disease Control 1987). Table 9.2 provides the CDCP's recommendations for HIV reporting and stresses the continued need for AIDS surveillance and HIV **sero-surveys**.

On January 1, 1993, the AIDS surveillance case definition for adolescents and adults was expanded beyond the definition established in 1987 to include all HIV-infected persons with severe immunosuppression, pulmonary tuberculosis, recurrent pneumonia, or invasive cancer (Centers for Disease Control 1994). As a result, the increase in the number of cases reported in 1993 (11 percent) exceeded the projected increase of 75 percent.

Sero-survey–a sero-survey involves seeking the presence of a particular antibody in the sera of an appropriately selected sample of the population. Surveys of seroimmunity are basic to the study of infectious diseases.

TABLE 9.2 Recommended Elements of HIV Infection Reporting

1. States requiring reports of HIV infection with or without personal identifiers should collect a minimum set of information to allow comparison of data beyond the state level. Reports should be collected in a manner that allows repeat positive reports to be excluded.
2. Data collected for HIV infection reporting (e.g., risk factor) should be consistent with data collected for other HIV activities such as AIDS case reporting and results from counseling and testing sites.
3. HIV infection reporting should be accompanied by appropriate safeguards for confidentiality to protect the individual and to reduce the potential negative impact on participation in voluntary counseling and testing activities.
4. CDC should collect summary data without personal identities and disseminate on a regular basis a minimum set of data from states with mandatory and voluntary reporting of HIV infection. Data include age, sex, race/ethnicity, state of residence, transmission category and clinical status.
5. HIV infection reporting should not interfere with AIDS case reprint or seroprevalence surveys. AIDS case reporting should be the primary means by which trends in incidence of HIV infection in the United States are followed.
6. HIV infection reporting should be evaluated rigorously to determine its usefulness in prevention programs and in monitoring trends. This evaluation needs to be conduced jointly by the states and CDC.

Source: From Centers for Disease Control. 1989. HIV Infection Reporting—United States. *Morbidity and Mortality Weekly Report* 38:496–499.

The surveillance information available as a result of the expanded AIDS reporting criteria provides a more complete estimate of (1) the number and distribution of persons with severe HIV-related immunosuppression and (2) the three major HIV-related illnesses that are important among groups in whom the growth of the AIDS epidemic has been the greatest.

Prevention

A person's risk of acquiring HIV infection through sexual contact depends on several factors: the number of different partners; the likelihood (prevalence) of HIV infection in these partners; and the probability of virus transmission during sexual contact with an infected partner (Peterman and Curran 1986). Given these factors, the risk of HIV infection is highest for a regular partner of an HIV-infected person.

An increase in other STDs among heterosexuals indicates the need for more intensive application of the recommended measures (Centers for Disease Control 1987) to interrupt the sexual and drug-use-related transmission of HIV infection. The measures include:

1. Development of community health education programs aimed at populations at increased risk

2. Participation in mutually monogamous relationships or reduction of the number of sex partners
3. Use of condoms to prevent exposure to semen and infected lymphocytes
4. Enrollment of drug users in programs to eliminate use of IV-drugs
5. Increased voluntary HIV testing and counseling of persons at increased risk in settings such as STD and family planning clinics and drug-treatment programs

The reduction of new HIV infections requires the cooperative efforts of public and private organizations.

Syphilis

Syphilis, a serious STD but far less common than chlamydia and gonorrhea, is caused by bacterium *treponema pallidum.* The bacteria easily penetrate the mucous membranes of the mouth, the vagina, and the penis' urethra. The incubation period lasts 2–3 weeks but can be as long as 8 weeks. This primary stage of syphilis begins with a hard, painless, red, protruding sore or ulcer called a chancre (pronounced "shanker"). The chancre can show up on the genitals, the rectum, and occasionally on the tongue; if the chancre is developing in the vagina or cervix, it can go unnoticed. The primary stage of syphilis also includes swelling of the lymph nodes nearest the chancre. A diagnosis can be made by a microscopic examination of the chancre's fluid.

After the chancre heals, then two to six weeks later, secondary syphilis begins. The symptoms can include general malaise, fever, headache, loss of appetite, joint pain, enlarged lymph nodes, and a non-itching skin rash of small red bumps. A diagnosis of secondary syphilis can be made by a blood test.

Late (latent) syphilis, the final stage, occurs three or more years after the initial contact with the bacteria. This stage flares up without warning, mimicking many chronic conditions. The heart and joints can be affected as well as the central nervous system, which can lead to paralysis, senility, and blindness. Untreated syphilis can also be given by a mother to her newborn. Congenital syphilis can be prevented by the appropriate treatment of the mother during pregnancy (Centers for Disease Control 1988).

Who Is at Risk?

In 1946 there were 94,957 reported U.S. cases of primary and secondary syphilis, with a steady decline to 6,392 reported cases in 1956. However, the number of cases rose sharply to 19,851 by 1961. As Table 9.3 indicates, the number of cases continued to increase until 1990, with a drop in cases reported in 1992. The increase in infectious syphilis in the past decade (Table 9.4) suggests an important shift in the epidemiological

TABLE 9.3 Reported Cases of Primary and Secondary Syphilis from 1983 to 1992—United States

Year	Number of Cases Primary and Secondary	Total All Stages
1983	32,698	74,637
1985	27,143	67,563
1987	35,241	86,545
1988	40,117	103,437
1990	50,223	134,255
1992	33,973	112,581

Source: Data from Centers for Disease Control. 1993. Summary of notifiable diseases, United States, 1992. *Morbidity and Mortality Weekly Report* 41:55.

TABLE 9.4 Incidence Rate of Primary and Secondary Syphilis > 7.0/100,000 and an Increase Between 1985 and 1988—United States

Area	1985		1988	
	No.	Rate	No.	Rate
District of Columbia	342	55.3	426	69.1
Florida	3,679	32.6	7,453	62.5
California	4,326	16.6	7,718	28.2
New York	2,530	14.2	5,004	28.1
Nevada	64	6.9	180	18.1
North Carolina	672	10.9	752	11.9
Oregon	112	4.2	310	11.4
Delaware	39	6.3	71	11.1
Connecticut	215	6.8	334	10.5
Pennsylvania	513	4.3	941	7.9
Total United States	27,143	11.5	35,241	14.6

Source: Data from Centers for Disease Control. 1988. Syphilis and congenital syphilis—United States, 1985–1988. *Morbidity and Mortality Weekly Report* 37:486–489.

pattern in the United States (Centers for Disease Control 1988). As infectious syphilis has decreased among homosexual and bisexual males, largely because of changes in sexual behavior due to AIDS, a sizable increase has occurred among heterosexuals (Table 9.5). A similar shift was documented earlier in two small outbreaks (Centers for Disease Control 1987; Lee et al. 1987).

The cause of this increase is unknown, but several hypotheses have been proposed. First, anecdotal reports from persons interviewing syphilis patients and their sexual partners indicate that prostitution, in which non-intravenous drugs (especially crack cocaine) are often exchanged for sex,

Epidemiology and Sexually Transmitted Diseases

TABLE 9.5 Cases of Primary and Secondary Syphilis, by Sexual Preference (Male)—United States, January–March 1986 and January–March 1987

Reporting Area/ Characteristic*	Number of Cases		
	January– March 1986	January– March 1987	Change (%)
California			
Sexual preference (male)**			
Heterosexual	643	1,130	(76)
Homosexual/bisexual	277	148	(–47)
New York City			
Sexual preference (male)*			
Heterosexual	125	250	(100)
Homosexual/bisexual	45	22	(–51)

Source: From Centers for Disease Control. 1987. Increases in primary and secondary syphilis—United States. *Morbidity and Mortality Weekly Report* 36:393–397.

*Demographic data were available for 99 percent of patients with reported cases.

**Excludes men whose sexual preference was not determined. These comprise 2 percent of men with syphilis in California and 53 percent in New York City.

may be partially responsible for the outbreaks of syphilis as well as other STDs (Rolfs, Goldberg, and Sharrar 1987).

Second, it has been suggested that the routine use of **spectinomycin** in geographical areas where a sizable proportion of gonorrhea infections are caused by **B-lactamase**-producing organisms may explain the increase in infectious syphilis since the gonococcus organism has developed a resistance to the antibiotic. Spectinomycin does not appear to cure incubating syphilis (Rein 1976). Third, the decrease in the resources available for syphilis control programs has been suggested as a contributing factor.

Increases in infectious syphilis among females and heterosexuals are of a concern for three reasons. First, an increase in the number of females with syphilis will probably be followed by increased morbidity and mortality from congenital syphilis. Second, the marked increase among inner-city, heterosexual minority groups suggests that high risk sexual activity is increasing in these groups despite the risk of HIV infection, which is already elevated because of the high prevalence of intravenous drug abuse (Centers for Disease Control 1988). Third, United States and African studies note that genital ulcer diseases, such as primary syphilis, increase the risk of HIV transmission (Quinn et. al., 1987; Cameron et al. 1987).

Prevention

The cause of fetal or perinatal death in approximately 40 percent of affected pregnancies (Centers for Disease Control 1988) is congenital

Spectinomycin– spectinomycin is an antimicrobial agent. Many bacteria and some fungi manifest resistance to antimicrobial agents. **B-lactamase–**certain bacteria are resistant to some penicillin and cephalosporin antibiotics that produce the enzyme beta lactamase. This enzyme binds to antibiotics that possess a beta lactam ring and opens the ring to activate the antibiotic.

syphilis, which is a preventable consequence of untreated syphilis in pregnant women. Congenital syphilis can be expected to continue to increase in frequency, because increases in congenital syphilis tend to lag behind increases in women by about one year (Centers for Disease Control 1988). Prevention measures need to address the likelihood that urban African-American and Hispanic women, who have had a disproportionate increase in the incidence of syphilis, are less likely than white women to receive early prenatal care (Ingram, Makuc, and Kleinman 1986).

It is clear that preventive measures against the spread of congenital syphilis need to include (1) syphilis screening of pregnant and childbearing-aged women to identify those who need treatment and (2) the removal of obstacles that prevent women from receiving early prenatal care, especially in areas with high syphilis incidence.

Finally, the interventions that are essential if the trend of increased syphilis rates are to be reversed need to focus on the following issues:

1. Reemphasizing the traditional methods of syphilis control—patient interviews and sex partner notification
2. Conducting screening for STDs in high risk populations
3. Assuring access to quality clinical care by removing financial barriers and other obstacles (e.g., long waiting times and lack of evening hours)
4. Enhancing the current surveillance systems to allow the ongoing evaluation of intervention strategies and effective resource allocation (Centers for Disease Control 1988)

Gonorrhea

After chlamydia, gonorrheal infection ranks the highest of STDs. The historical reporting of cases of gonorrhea is described in Table 9.6. However, the true number of reported gonorrhea cases may be actually higher due to underreporting cases from the private health sector.

Gonorrhea is caused by the *neisseria gonorrhoeae* bacterium. The incidence of antibiotic–resistant gonorrhea continues to increase each year and is spreading to previously unaffected geographical areas. A specific diagnosis of gonorrhea requires a culture. With men, however, a physician can usually make an accurate diagnosis on the basis of symptoms and a microscopic examination of the urethra's puslike discharge. In women, the vagina's many bacterial secretions can resemble gonorrhea under the microscope, so a culture is recommended.

Who Is at Risk?

During the 1980s, substantial declines in the occurrence of gonorrhea among homosexual and bisexual men was documented in the United States (Judson 1983). It is believed that these trends reflect changes in sexual behavior in response to the epidemic of AIDS (Handfield 1985).

TABLE 9.6 Number of Reported Cases of Gonorrhea from 1969 to 1992—United States

Year	Number of Cases
1969	534,872
1971	670,268
1973	842,621
1975	999,937
1977	1,002,219
1979	1,004,058
1981	990,864
1983	900,435
1985	911,419
1987	780,905
1988	719,536
1989	700,751
1992	501,409

Source: Data from Centers for Disease Control. 1993. Summary of notifiable disease, United States, 1992. *Morbidity and Mortality Weekly Report* 42:RR14.

Many people carry the bacterium and have no signs of illness. Thus, a pregnant woman can unknowingly pass the disease to her baby during delivery. The disease then often attacks the infant's eyes and may cause blindness. Consequently, prophylactic eye drops of 1-percent **silver nitrate solution** are given to newborn infants as a standard public health measure.

Women are at risk for **pelvic inflammatory disease** (PID), the major complication of a gonorrheal infection. If untreated, gonorrhea can spread through the bloodstream and infect the body's organs. PID is a major cause of infertility. PID occurs in about 15 percent of women when the bacteria proceed from the cervix to infect the fallopian tubes.

Those who engage in oral or anal sex with gonorrhea-infected persons can become infected in the mouth, throat, and rectum. Usually mild symptoms, like a sore throat and tonsillitis, occur. Signs of anal gonorrhea are a constant urge to move the bowels, with an associated purulent discharge.

Prevention

The challenge for sexually active homosexual and bisexual males, as the incidence of STDs and HIV infections declines, is to not relax behaviors regarding sexual safety. Maintaining life-style changes such as abstinence or monogamy may become more difficult with time and "risky sexual relapse" could occur (Elkstrand et al. 1989).

With the increasing proportion of gonorrhea in the United States caused by antibiotic-resistant strains of *neisseria gonorrhoeae* surveillance, patient care, and outbreak management procedures must be in place to

Silver nitrate solutions–these are used therapeutically as germicides. One drop of a 1-percent solution of silver nitrate is placed in the eyes of newborn babies to prevent gonorrheal infections. **Pelvic inflammatory disease**–pelvic inflammatory disease (salpingitis) occurs when infectious agents invade the uterus and spread to the fallopian tubes, ovaries, and surrounding tissues.

identify new cases rapidly in order to limit transmission. In addition, the design of control efforts need to include (1) available resources; (2) total and "at-risk" population sizes and characteristics; (3) the travel patterns of infected individuals; and (4) the proximity of the locality to known endemic areas (Centers for Disease Control 1987).

Chlamydia

Nonspecific Urethritis–nonspecific urethritis (NSU), or nongonococcal urethritis, is a common sexually transmitted disease. It is an infection of the urethra. About half of the cases of NSU are caused by the chlamydia organism.

Chlamydia (pronounced klah-MID-e-a) is an STD caused by a virus-like bacterium called *chlamydia trachomatis*. It is sometimes labeled as "nongonococcal urethritis" or NSU **(nonspecific urethritis).** This disease attacks the reproductive system and often displays no symptoms, eventually leading to painful pelvic inflammation, miscarriages, and infertility. When symptoms are present, they are usually painful urination, abdominal pain, and bleeding between menstrual periods. Chlamydia has been labeled as the "invisible disease" and is estimated to infect about five million people in the United States. The total number of chlamydia cases ranks the highest of the known STDs (Table 9.7).

Who Is at Risk?

Chlamydia is most often contracted by young heterosexuals. This disease may live undetected in either the female or male genital tract for as long as eight years.

Newborns can become infected if their mothers have chlamydia; the infants then develop eye infections or pneumonia. In males, chlamydia can cause infections of the urethra and possibly sterility.

Surveillance

In the past, the only method to diagnose chlamydia was to culture the bacteria, a process that took several days. Testing for chlamydia has been time consuming, expensive, and in some communities simply unavailable. We

TABLE 9.7 Estimated New Cases of Sexually Transmitted Diseases— United States, 1990

Disease	Number of New Cases/Year
AIDS	80,000
Syphilis	100,000
Herpes	200,000–500,000
Gonorrhea	2,000,000
Chlamydia	5,000,000

Source: From Centers for Disease Control. 1990. *Morbidity and Mortality Weekly Report* 39:321–330.

Epidemiology and Sexually Transmitted Diseases

know, however, that early detection is important to prevent chronic effects. Now there are several inexpensive tests physicians can use. Chlamydia, until recent years, was not a notifiable disease for which the CDCP collected universal data. Many states by virtue of mandatory health regulations, have listed chlamydia as a reportable disease. Chlamydia is considered by some researchers as having been lost in the shuffle for resources since the mid-1980s funding of AIDS projects. Greater surveillance is needed to assess more accurately the actual size of this silent epidemic.

Prevention

Curing chlamydia, once it is correctly diagnosed, is relatively simple and inexpensive. With early discovery, the bacteria can be killed with antibiotic treatment. Some experts believe the most effective ways to stop the spread of chlamydia are to do the following:

1. Set up voluntary screening of high risk groups, which would generally include sexually active individuals who have multiple or new partners.
2. Conduct more chlamydia-related research studies.
3. Educate consumers to be more careful in their choice of sexual partners and to use barrier methods, such as the condom and the diaphragm, to reduce transmission of the infection.
4. Advise women to be tested for chlamydia before they become pregnant.

Summary

This chapter reviewed the basic factors in risk control for AIDS and other sexually transmitted diseases. In addition, surveillance, prevention and intervention strategies were discussed. The underlying tenet of this chapter is that a healthy life-style depends in many ways on the amount of risk each one of us undertakes in daily living. Risk control can begin with acquiring knowledge of the sexually transmitted diseases. Health-care providers play a critical role in motivating individuals to accept responsibility for their own health and others'.

The frequency of each STD is not constant within the population. It is important for health workers to understand the reasons for the changing epidemiological patterns of sexually transmitted diseases in the United States and other countries.

Discussion Questions

1. Check with your state department of public health to see if the gonorrhea rate has increased since last year. If the gonorrhea rate has increased, what public health interventions do you suggest to

reverse the increased trend? If the gonorrhea rate has declined, what accounts for the decline?

2. Develop your own "AIDS myth-fact sheet."
3. Identify the AIDS-related community resources currently in place in the following locations: (a) your home town (community level), (b) the campus, (c) your state of residence (state level), and (d) the United States (federal level).
4. Describe the basic stages of untreated syphilis.
5. What interventions may be employed by public health personnel to combat syphilis?
6. Who are at greatest risk for developing gonorrhea?
7. Why is chlamydia called the "invisible disease"?

References

Beneson, A. S. (ed) 1990. Control of communicable diseases in man. 15th ed. Washington, D.C.: American Public Health Association.

Cameron, D. W., F. Plummer, J. N. Simonson et al. 1987. Female to male heterosexual transmission of HIV infection in Nairobi. Presented at the International Society for STD Research, Atlanta, GA, August 2–5, 1987.

Centers for Disease Control. 1987. Antibiotic-resistant strains of neisseria gonorrhoeae: Policy guidelines for detection, management and control. 36:5S.

———. 1987. Classification system for human immunodeficiency virus (HIV) infection in children under 13 years of age. *Morbidity and Mortality Weekly Report* 36:225–230, 236.

———. 1988. Continuing increase in infectious syphilis—United States. *Morbidity and Mortality Weekly Report* 37:35–38.

———. 1987. Early syphilis—Broward County Florida. *Morbidity and Mortality Weekly Report* 36:221–223.

———. 1988. Guidelines for the prevention and control of congenital syphilis. *Morbidity and Mortality Weekly Report* 37 (supplement S–1).

———. 1994. Heterosexually acquired AIDS—United States, 1993. *Morbidity and Mortality Weekly Report* 43(9):155–159.

———. 1991. Mortality attributable to HIV infection/AIDS—United States, 1981–1990. *Morbidity and Mortality Weekly Report* 40:121–125.

———. 1987. Public Health Service guidelines for counseling and antibody testing to prevent HIV infection and AIDS. *Morbidity and Mortality Weekly Report* 36:509–515, 521–522.

———. 1993. Summary of notifiable disease, United States. *Morbidity and Mortality Weekly Report* 41:55.

———. 1988. Syphilis and congenital syphilis—United States, 1985–1988. *Morbidity and Mortality Weekly Report* 37:486–489.

———. 1994. Update. Impact of the expanded AIDS surveillance case definition for adolescents and adults on case reporting—United States, 1993. *Morbidity and Mortality Weekly Report* 43(9):160–171.

———. 1993. World AIDS day. *Morbidity and Mortality Weekly Report* 42:869.

———. 1992. Years of potential life lost before age 65—United States, 1992. *Morbidity and Mortality Weekly Report* 38:27–39.

Elkstrand, M. L., R. D. Stall, T. J. Coates, and L. McKusick. 1989. Risky sex relapse, the next challenge for AIDS prevention programs: The AIDS behavioral research project (abstract). 5th International Conference on AIDS, Montreal, June 4–9, 1989, p. 669.

Handfield, H. H. 1985. Decreasing incidence of gonorrhea in homosexually active men—minimal effect on risk of AIDS. *Western Journal of Medicine* 143:469–470.

Holmes, K., J. Karon, and J. Kaeiss. 1990. The increasing frequency of heterosexually acquired AIDS in the United States. *American Journal of Public Health* 80:858–862.

Ingram, D. D., D. Makuc, and J. C. Kleinman. 1986. National and state trends in use of prenatal care 1970–73. *American Journal of Public Health* 76:415–423.

Judson, F. N. 1983. Fear of AIDS and gonorrhea rates in homosexual men. *Lancet* 2:159–160.

Karin, L. 1989. AIDS prevention and chemical dependence treatment needs of women and their children. *Journal of Psychoactive Drugs* 21:396–399.

Lee, C. B., R. C. Brunham, E. Sherman, and G. K. M. Harding. 1987. Epidemiology of an outbreak of infectious syphilis in Manitoba. *American Journal of Epidemiology* 125:227–283.

National Center for Health Statistics. 1993. Annual summary of births, marriages, divorces and deaths: United States, 1992. *Monthly Vital Statistics Report* 41(13). Hyattsville, MD: U.S. Department of Health and Human Services.

Peterman, T. A., and J. W. Curran. 1986. Sexual transmission of human immunodeficiency virus. *Journal of the American Medical Association* 256:2222–2226.

Quinn, S. 1993. AIDS and the African-American woman: The triple burden of race, class, and gender. *Health Education Quarterly* 20(3):306–320.

Quinn, T. C., D. Glassner, D. L. Matuszak et. al. 1987. Screening for human immunodeficiency virus (HIV) infection of patients attending sexually transmitted diseases clinics: Risk factors and correlates of infection. Presented at the International Society for STD Research, Atlanta, GA, August 2–5, 1987.

Rein, M. F. 1976. Biopharmacology of syhilotherapy. *Journal of American Venereal Disease Association* 3:107–127.

Rolfs, R. T., M. Goldberg, and R. G. Sharrar. 1987. Outbreak of early syphilis in Philadelphia. Presented at the 115th Annual Meeting of American Public Health Association, New Orleans, LA, October 18–22, 1987.

CHAPTER 10

Foodborne Disease

Introduction

Although the term "food poisoning" is generally applied to any disease caused by food, the more appropriate name is *foodborne illness.* This rubric includes not only true poisonings, such as those from metabolic products (toxins) produced by certain microorganisms while they multiply in food (e.g., staphylococcus aureus), but also foodborne "infections" such as salmonellosis.

The potential for large-scale foodborne outbreaks still exists due to the increasing reliance on the massive processing, production, and distribution of food to our population. Thus, any contamination in that chain could result in the exposure of large numbers of people to foodborne disease.

The Centers for Disease Control and Prevention defines an outbreak as "an incident in which two or more persons experience a similar illness after ingestion of a common food, and epidemiologic analysis implicates the food as the source of the illness" (Centers for Disease Control 1992). There are, however, two exceptions to this definition in that one case of botulism or chemical poisoning also constitutes a foodborne outbreak.

In recent years, about five hundred outbreaks have been reported annually in the United States. In only about 40 percent of these was a cause identified. Of those foodborne outbreaks in which a cause was identified, 75 percent of the cases were of bacterial origin, 20 percent were chemical, 3 percent were parasitic, and 2 percent were viral. Most outbreaks of bacterial origin involve salmonella, staphylccoccus, and clostridium perfringens. Table 10.1 shows the distinctive features of these three common causes of foodborne illness. The data presented in Table 10.1 display the different clinical features and incubation periods of each illness. These are important in investigating a foodborne outbreak, because they enable investigators to make a judgment as to a probable cause early in an epidemiological investigation. Specifically, this knowledge can help investigators determine how far back in time they should inquire about food exposures.

TABLE 10.1 Distinctive Features of the Three Most Common Bacterial Causes of Foodborne Illness

Illness	Incubation Period (In Hours)	Fever	Vomiting	Diarrhea
Staphylococcal poisoning	3	No	Yes	Yes/No
Clostridium perfringens poisoning	12	No	No	Yes
Salmonella infection	24	Yes	Yes/No	Yes

Source: Adapted from Werner, S. In "Food Poisoning," *Public health and preventive medicine*, ed. J. Last and R. Wallace. Norwalk, CT: Appleton and Lange, 1992.

Each year approximately 9,100 people die from foodborne illness in the United States (Centers for Disease Control 1990). At greater risk of death from such illnesses are children, the elderly, and those individuals with compromised immune systems. In the United States, between one and ten billion dollars are spent annually on foodborne illness, which includes days lost from work and medical expenses (Marshall 1988).

When one buys a steak at a grocery store, the estimated risk is one in twenty that it will contain bacteria. For pork, the risk is one in eight, and higher still is chicken with a one in three risk. Many experts believe that most of the contamination occurs at the time of initial processing. The potential is great for bacteria to escape from the animal's feces as the carcass is butchered. The exposure of the intestines during processing is another source of contamination.

The lack of strong statistical evidence of the increase in outbreaks encourages some officials to blame illness rates on consumers (Marshall 1988). They might cite, for example, toxicity that is due to food handling practices in the home, restaurants, and other facilities. Proper cooking will kill virtually all harmful agents, with few exceptions, such as enterotoxins (poisons affecting the gastrointestinal tract that are found in food contaminated by staphylococci organisms). The new Food and Drug Administration Code now has uniform food sanitation standards for industry and all establishments that produce or handle food. In addition, there is also an emphasis on applying HACCPs (Hazard Analysis Critical Control Points) at the industrial and local level in order to control possible contamination or the conditions that allow the survival and/or growth of bacteria or other organisms.

Surveillance and Investigation

The surveillance of foodborne diseases is generally aimed at disease control through (1) the identification and removal of contaminated products from the commercial market; (2) the identification and correction of improper food handling practices in commercial establishments and in the home; and (3) the identification and treatment of cases and carriers of foodborne disease. Furthermore, surveillance also contributes to our knowledge of disease causation and new agents and their food vehicles (Werner 1992).

Generally, in relatively small outbreaks, an investigator should attempt to question all persons who were exposed, whether ill or not, for symptoms and food consumed. In order to identify the contaminated food, a method similar to a cohort study design is commonly used (see Chapter 8). The rates of illness in those persons who ate specific food items are calculated and compared with the rates of illness in those who did not eat the items. The implicated foods have the highest attack rates. When the rates for eaters and noneaters are compared, the implicated foods display the greatest differences in attack rates. Such differences are called the "attributable risk" or the rate of disease that can be attributed to the food under consideration. In Table 10.2, barbecued chicken appears to be the implicated food item. Note, though, that more ill and well people consumed iced tea than any other item, reflecting the popularity of the drink. The necessity of interviewing well people in order to incriminate a particular food is illustrated by the iced tea item.

One might assume that the association of illness with a particular implicated food should be almost perfect in that all those who ate the item would have become ill. However, Werner (1992) states that there are several reasons why this rarely happens:

1. The implicated food may not be contaminated throughout.
2. Host susceptibility varies.
3. Dosage (the quantity consumed) varies.
4. Food histories may contain reporting errors through faulty recall, uncertainty, or lying; there may also be errors in recording.
5. Those who report illness but no exposure to the incriminated food may have a coincidental, unrelated illness or secondary infection when the outbreak is due to infection (e.g., salmonella); alternatively, illness may be due to trace contamination of other foods or utensils by the implicated food.

When foodborne outbreaks occur in a relatively large population, so that it is not feasible to interview all the participants, a random sample can be selected and questioned for food exposure history and symptoms. The collected data can also be assembled in a prospective manner and similarly analyzed as in Table 10.2.

Before the true nature of **foodborne illness** can be determined and control measures carried out, the surveillance of these illnesses must be intensified. Foodborne disease **surveillance** requires: knowing why the

Foodborne intoxication–a generic term applied to illnesses acquired through the consumption of contaminated food or water. The term applies to intoxications caused by chemical contaminants (heavy metals and others); and toxins from bacterial growth (staphylococcus aureus, clostridium botulinum). They may also be acquired from a variety of organic substances that may be present in natural foods, such as certain mushrooms, mussels, fish, and other seafood. This definition also includes acute foodborne infections such as salmonellosis.

Surveillance of disease–the continuing scrutiny of all aspects of the occurrence and spread of disease that are pertinent to effective control.

TABLE 10.2 Differences in Food Specific Attack Rates in an Outbreak of Foodborne Illness

Food	Persons Who Ate Specified Food				Persons Who Did Not Eat Specified Food				Difference in Attack Rate
	Ill	Well	Total	Attack Rate %	Ill	Well	Total	Attack Rate %	
Shrimp	8	4	12	67	15	21	36	42	+25
Fried chicken	10	33	43	23	4	2	6	67	−44
Baked beans	12	13	25	48	12	10	22	55	−7
Barbecued chicken	17	1	18	94	3	27	30	10	+84
Potato salad	17	20	37	46	8	6	14	57	−11
Iced tea	23	23	46	50	0	2	2	0	+50
Bread	8	9	17	47	18	13	31	58	−11
Ice cream	1	2	3	33	21	21	42	50	−17

Source: Adapted from Werner, S. In Last, J. and Wallace, R. (Eds.) *Public health and preventive medicine.* Norwalk, CT: Appleton and Lange, 1992.

illnesses are reported; investigating outbreaks; obtaining laboratory confirmation of sporadic cases; interpreting data; and disseminating the resultant facts.

If epidemiologists are able to pinpoint early the food responsible for an outbreak of foodborne illness, then immediate action can be taken. Control measures include stopping the sale of a particular food and distribution and recalling a contaminated food that has already been distributed. An example of a foodborne illness occurred in Cook County, Illinois, during October 1–3, 1990. In this outbreak, 534 (23 percent) of 1,900 persons from thirty states attending a convention banquet in Chicago became ill. Thirty attendees suffered **gastroenteritis** and sought medical treatment. Of the 435 ill persons, 147 (43 percent) were hospitalized. Cultures from 245 persons yielded **salmonella enteritidis**.

The Chicago Department of Health obtained case histories from 92 ill and 55 well persons who attended the banquet. Bread pudding with vanilla sauce was implicated as the most likely vehicle for the salmonella enteritidis. Of the 92 ill persons, 89 (97 percent) ate the pudding, compared with 24 (44 percent) of the 55 well persons. No other foods were associated with the illness. The implicated dessert was prepared with grade AA shell eggs and may have been undercooked. In addition, the dessert was left at room temperature for one to four hours between cooking and serving.

The eggs were traced to one specific farm, and salmonella enteritidis isolated from environmental samples of all six chicken houses tested positive. The sale of fresh eggs from this farm was restricted, and all eggs from the six houses were subsequently pasteurized (Centers for Disease Control 1990).

Gastroenteritis–a generic term, this is an inflammation of the stomach and intestinal tract. Certain diseases of known bacterial, viral, parasitic, or toxic etiology can be included in a clinical definition. Bacterial gastroenteritis includes cholera, salmonellosis and shigellosis.
Salmonella enteritidis–a type of bacteria causing gastroenteritis and food poisoning in humans. More than fourteen hundred species of salmonella have been classified.

As the Chicago example shows, investigating an outbreak requires the gathering of information about the hosts, the disease-causing agents, and their environments. Questions about the hosts and their environment begin with *what, when, where, who* and *why*. Questions about the agent and its environment begin with *what, where, how* and *why* (Table 10.3).

We know that the primary purpose of investigating an outbreak of possible foodborne illness is to gather information for prevention and control. In order to do this, epidemiologists need to know more then just a description of the disease and the source of the causative organism. They need to answer the following questions as well: Which factors allowed the organisms to survive in contaminated foods? Which factors permitted these organisms to multiply?

What We Do Affects Our Food

The way we heat, refrigerate, or handle food may have an effect on foodborne illness. The known factors contributing to foodborne illness outbreaks include the following:

1. Failing to refrigerate potentially hazardous foods
2. Allowing food to remain warm (at bacterial incubation temperatures)
3. Preparing foods several hours or days before intended use or using leftovers (with inadequate storage after preparation)
4. Failing to thoroughly cook or heat process contaminated food
5. Using a contaminated raw ingredient in a food that is to be served uncooked
6. Bringing contaminated raw foods containing organisms into the kitchen and **cross contaminating** cooked foods
7. Obtaining food supplies from unsafe sources
8. Failing to clean and disinfect kitchen utensils and equipment
9. Using utensils and serveware that contain toxic materials
10. Using poor dry storage practices

Cross contamination– occurs after a person touches a surface where an infectious agent is present and subsequently carries the agent to another surface. Cross contamination can occur when equipment is used to prepare contaminated raw food and then the same equipment is used for cooked foods.

In addition, precautions should be taken to prevent establishing environmental conditions that selectively permit pathogens to grow, while inhibiting competing organisms. In the Chicago example, the incompletely cooked eggs in the pudding held at room temperature before serving enabled the salmonella organism to grow to a higher concentration. An important environmental factor involved encouraging workers to wash their hands after each use of the toilet facilities. Food handlers, who may or may not have disease or skin sores, need to practice good personal hygiene, such as handwashing, so as to limit the transmission of disease. There are many other foodborne pathogens, and they may be transmitted by infected workers in a number of ways (Table 10.4).

TABLE 10.3 Factors to Discover in a Foodborne Disease Investigation

Agent	Environment (of Agent)	Environment (of Host)	Host
Type (*what*)	Source (*where*)	Human ecology (*why*)	Verify diagnosis (*what*)
Bacteria	Human	Biological	Symptoms
Rickettsiae	Animal	Chemical	Duration
Viruses	Fomites	Physical	Severity
Protozoa		Cultural	Incubation periods
Fungi	Contamination (*how*)	Socioeconomic	Specimens
Nematodes	Infected animal		Infectivity
Cestodes	Soil	Control (*what to do*)	
Trematodes	Feces to carcasses	Agent	Descriptive epidemiology
Algae	Raw ingredients	Refrigeration	Time (*when*)
Toxicants in plants	Infected worker (feces, nose,	Thorough cooking	of onset
and animals	throat, infection, skin)	or thermal	of eating
Chemicals	Preparation or processing	processing	of year
	method	Hot holding	Place (*where*)
Nature (*why*)	Equipment	Sanitation	of residence
Numbers		Safe storage	of eating
Toxigenicity	Vehicle (*what*)	People	of food source
Sporeformer	Food history attack rates	Personal hygiene	Person (*who*)
Theormostable	Samples	Carrier control	Age
Growth range	History of preparation	Immunization	Sex
Optimum growth	Source	(typhoid)	Foods eaten
Aerobic		Surveillance	Food preferences
Anaerobic	Survival, growth, and	Supervision	Occupation
Facultative	multiplication (*how*)	Training	Ethnic groups
Nutrients	Times	Equipment	Socioeconomic
pH range	Storage upon arrival	Construction	group
State of maturity	Preparation	Maintenance	Other factors
Concentration	Cooking or thermal	Different for raw	Compare with
Residence	processing	and prepared	control
Water activity	Storage during serving	foods	
	Chilling		
	Reheating		
	Storage after reheating		
	Storage before/after sampling		

Source: Bryan, F. L. 1982. *Diseases transmitted by foods: A classification and summary,* 2nd Ed., Atlanta: HHS Pub. No. (CDC) 83–8237, USPHS, Centers for Disease Control.

We have noted earlier that one of the most important parts of an epidemiological investigation is a careful review of the site where foods were processed or prepared. This is known as a *field investigation.* Sometimes a field investigation reveals a history of recent acute illness among the food handlers closely associated with a suspect meal or food. In such instances, the food handlers need to have physical examinations and to submit bodily specimens, depending on the illness present (Table 10.5).

We have already indicated a number of factors related to sources of contamination or to conditions that affect bacterial survival or growth.

TABLE 10.4 Sources of Transmission of Foodborne Pathogens by Infected Workers

Source	Mode of Transmission	Example Disease
Feces	Intestinal carriers who are excreting organisms, touch feces or contaminated skin with hands, fail to wash hands adequately, and subsequently handle food before organisms succumb to drying or the pH reaction of the skin.	Typhoid fever; Paratyphoid fever; Salmonellosis; Shigellosis; Infectious hepatitis; *c. perfringens* foodborne illness; Enterococcal foodborne illness; Enteropathogenic *E. coli* infections.
Infected lesions	Workers touch food with infected lesion, or they touch lesion with hands and then handle foods.	Staphylococcal intoxication; Beta hemolytic streptococcal infection.
Nose or throat	Workers touch food with infected lesion, or they touch lesion with hands and then handle foods.	Staphylococcal intoxication; Beta hemolytic streptococcal infection
Raw foods of animal origin	Workers touch raw foods or equipment that previously contacted raw foods and then handle other foods.	

Source: Bryan, F. L. 1982. *Diseases transmitted by foods: A classification and summary.* 2nd Ed. Atlanta: HHS Pub. No. (CDC) 83–8237. USPHS, Centers for Disease Control.

TABLE 10.5 Specimen Needed for Suspected Illness

Suspected Illness	Specimen from Food Worker
Beta hemolytic streptococcal infections	Throat, anterior nasal; nasopharyngeal; septic lesions or pus
C. perfringens foodborne illness	Stool or rectal swab
Enterococcal infections	Stool or rectal swab
Enteropathogenic E. Coli	Stool or rectal swab
Parasitic infections	Stool
Salmonellosis	Stool or rectal swab; blood (on rare occasions)
Shigellosis	Stool or rectal swab
Staphylococcal intoxication	Anterior nasal; nasopharyngeal; septic lesion or pus; skin surface swab, hand swab, or rinse
Typhoid fever	Stool; blood; urine

Source: Bryan, F. L. 1982. *Diseases transmitted by foods: A classification and summary.* 2nd Ed.

Additional factors that might contribute to food illness outbreaks include the following (Benenson 1990):

1. Initial numbers of contaminating organisms
2. Types of organisms present in food
3. Microbial competition
4. Moisture and salt or sugar concentration (water activity)
5. Nutrients (type of food)
6. Oxygen tension and oxidation–reduction potential in the food
7. pH level
8. Presence of inhibitory substances
9. Physical state and biological structure of the food

Altering some factors to control the growth of organisms may produce a selective environment, inhibiting the growth of some bacteria but permitting others to grow. Vacuum packing, for instance, inhibits the growth of many bacteria, but C. botulinum can grow well in vacuum-packed food. Salt inhibits many organisms but not staphylococci (Frazier and Westhoff 1978).

Bacterial Diseases

Foodborne disease can be classified on the basis of the type of agent responsible for the illness. The types of agents are: bacterial, viral, and rickettsial; parasitic (cestodes, helminths, nematodes, protozoan, trematodes); fungal (mushroom or mycotoxin); poisonous plants and chemicals; and radionuclides and toxic animals.

In this and the following sections, we will look at selected foodborne diseases from bacterial, parasitic, and viral agents. We begin with bacterial diseases.

Clostridium

Causative Organisms.   Clostridium perfringens Type A is the cause of typical foodborne outbreaks in developed countries. The soil and the gastrointestinal tract of healthy persons and animals (cattle, pigs, poultry, and fish) serve as the main reservoirs of the bacteria. Most often, the implicated food is a meat dish that was contaminated by soil or feces and then held under conditions that allowed the organism to multiply. Almost all clostridium outbreaks have been associated with inadequately cooked meats in which the spores have survived normal cooking temperatures and have germinated as soon as the cooling period reached a suitable temperature. Foodborne outbreaks of clostridium are most often traced to food catering firms, restaurants, cafeterias, and schools.

Incubation Period.   The incubation period has a range of 6–24 hours, with a median of approximately 12 hours. The symptoms include acute abdominal cramps, diarrhea, and occasional dehydration and prostration. The duration of the illness is only about one day or less, and rarely are nausea, vomiting, fever, or chills present. In most cases, the disease is so mild that medical attention is rarely sought. In elderly debilitated patients, however, the disease can be severe and deaths have been reported (Werner 1992).

Control Measures. In order to avoid clostridium, meat dishes should be served either hot or at a temperature below 40°F. The meat may be served cold, but if it is to be served hot, it should be rewarmed to 165°F as quickly as possible. The expression "keep hot foods hot and cold foods cold" is worth emphasizing for most organisms responsible for foodborne disease. Good personal hygiene must also be practiced, and sewage must be disposed of in a sanitary manner.

Salmonellosis

Causative Organisms. Over two thousand serotypes exist but only about two hundred are detected in the United States in a given year. In most outbreaks, only a small number of serotypes account for the majority of confirmed cases of illness. S. typhimurium and S. enteritidis are the most common types reported.

Domestic and wild animals, including poultry, swine, cattle, rodents, turtles, dogs, cats; convalescent carriers; and mild and unrecognized cases serve as reservoirs. The agent is transmitted by the ingestion of organisms in food contaminated by feces of an infected animal or person. Fecal-oral transmission from person to person is important when diarrhea is present. Epidemics of salmonellosis are generally traced to commercially processed meat products, inadequately cooked poultry and poultry products, raw or undercooked eggs, or foods contaminated with feces by an infected food handler. Contaminated utensils and work surfaces also serve as sources of contamination. It is estimated that only 1 percent of clinical cases are reported in the United States each year, even though five million are thought to have salmonellosis during the year (Werner 1992).

Incubation Period. Usually symptoms appear within 12–36 hours, but onset varies from 6–72 hours. For several days there can be diarrhea, abdominal pain, chills, fever, vomiting, dehydration, anorexia, and headache.

Control Measures. At the point of production, proper farm sanitation should be maintained, protecting food and feed from animal, human, bird, insect, and rodent excreta. Animal feeds and all ingredients should be heat-treated. Meat and poultry need to be processed in a sanitary manner, and equipment should be sanitized. Food handlers should wash their hands after touching raw meat and avoid cross contamination from raw to cooked foods. Foods must be thoroughly cooked and chilled rapidly in small quantities if stored.

Staphylococcal Intoxication (Staphylococcus Food Poisoning)

Causative Organisms. The agent of staphylococcal food poisoning involves one of several **enterotoxins** of staphylococcus aureus which are stable at boiling temperature. This type of foodborne illness usually occurs by the host ingesting a food product containing staphylococcal enterotoxins. Unlike salmonellae, staphylococci are not normally classified as intestinal organisms but thrive, instead, in the mucous areas of the human nose and mouth, on the skin, in pimples, in skin lesions, and under the fingernails. In contaminated protein foods the organisms reproduce to dangerous quantities in four or more hours, depending on the temperature. The enterotoxin is thermostable and thus is not destroyed by heat. Therefore, any food that contains the enterotoxin needs to be destroyed.

Enterotoxin–toxins produced in or originating in the intestinal contents. Certain bacteria can produce enterotoxin which causes symptoms characteristic of food poisoning.

Incubation Period. There is a sudden onset of nausea in about 2–4 hours with a range of 1–6 hours. Other symptoms include excessive salivation, vomiting, diarrhea, abdominal cramps, and dehydration, as well as sweating, weakness, and prostration. The duration of the illness is short, lasting not more than a day or two, usually without fever.

Control Measures. The major requirements for producing sufficient enterotoxin to cause disease are that (1) the food must be contaminated with enterotoxin-producing staphylococci; (2) the food must be a good growth medium such as a high protein food; and (3) the food must be held at an improper temperature (45° to 115°F) for several hours.

Prevention primarily depends on safe food handling practices; excluding food handlers with purulent discharges, common colds, etc.; minimizing actual food handling time; and keeping food hot (above 140°F) or cold (below 40°F) and covered to exclude dust.

Parasitic Diseases

Trichinosis

Causative Organism. Trichinella spiralis, a delicate threadlike roundworm (nematode) is the causative organism. The larvae is ingested, and the female parasitic worms invade the mucosa of the small intestine. There they deposit larvae, which travel via the blood stream and lymphatic system of the body to be encysted into the muscle tissue.

Myocarditis–an inflammation of the middle layer of the walls of the heart.
Eosinophile–any of the white blood cells that are stainable with a dye that increase greatly in number in certain allergic and parasitic diseases.

Incubation Period. It usually takes about 9 days, with a range of 4–28 days, for incubation to occur. During the first stage (intestinal invasion), nausea, vomiting, diarrhea, and abdominal pain are present. In the second stage (muscle penetration), there is irregular and persistent fever, edema of the eyes, profuse sweating, muscular pain, thirst, skin lesions, chills, prostration, and labored breathing. Finally, in the third stage (tissue repair), there is generalized toxemia, **myocarditis**, and a higher **eosinophile** blood count.

Control Measures.   To control trichinosis, rodents should be eliminated from hog lots and garbage for feeding pigs should be cooked at 212°F for thirty minutes. The butchered pork must be adequately cured. Pork should be cooked thoroughly (until it turns white) or to 171°F or more. Pork should be frozen and stored in less than six-inch cuts at 5°F for twenty days, –10°F for ten days and –20°F for six days. Pork cuts greater than six inches thick should be stored at 5°F for thirty days, –10°F for twenty days, and at –20°F for twelve days.

Viral Diseases

Hepatitis A (Infectious Hepatitis)

Causative Organism.   Hepatitis virus A (virus of infectious hepatitis) is the causative agent, which survives freezing and retains its infectivity in feces for at least 2 weeks. It is completely inactivated by heating at 100°C for 5 minutes

Incubation Period.   Incubation usually occurs within 25–30 days, with a range of 14–50 days. This systemic infection causes gastrointestinal problems and injury to the liver. The symptoms include fever, anorexia, malaise, nausea, abdominal discomfort, bile in the urine, and a jaundiced skin color. The illness can last from a few weeks to several months and is usually more severe as age increases.

Control Measures.   Measures include disposing of sewage safely, preventing shellfish growing areas from sewage contamination, and treating water by coagulation, settling, filtration, and chlorination. Personal hygiene must be practiced and foods need to be cooked thoroughly. Persons with the disease need to be isolated for seven to ten days after jaundice occurs. Gama globulin should be given to those who have had contacts with an infected person. All needles, syringes, and other medical instruments used for parenteral injections (outside the intestines) must be well sterilized.

Summary

The potential for large scale foodborne outbreaks has never been greater. A major reason for increased surveillance is our greater reliance on massive, centralized food production and processing combined with extensive distribution. Any contamination in that chain could result in exposure of thousands, whereas contamination of foods processed in the home, exposes relatively few individuals. Technological advances in food production, distribution, and processing to the consumer have not always been coupled with advances that assured food safety.

This chapter has discussed the importance of food surveillance and investigation of the major foodborne diseases that affect our society. The prevention of foodborne illness is everyone's responsibility. Public health officials have the added responsibility of conducting thorough surveillance of reported illnesses. A quality investigation requires the stringent application of the "what, when, where, who and why" questioning format.

The basic precautions for avoiding foodborne illness outbreaks need to be understood and practiced by everyone. As individuals become familiar with some of the foodborne diseases, this will hopefully engender preventive behaviors.

Discussion Questions

1. Define a foodborne illness.
2. Why doesn't everyone who ingests a contaminated food item become ill?
3. Describe the major factors that contribute to foodborne illness outbreaks.
4. Identify the major types of agents responsible for foodborne illness.
5. Distinguish between salmonellosis and and staphylococcal foodborne illness.
6. Describe the major mode of transmission for salmonellosis and staphylococcal foodborne illnesses.

References

Benenson, A. S. 1990. *Control of communicable diseases in men*, 15th ed. Washington, D.C.: American Public Health Association.

Centers for Disease Control. 1992. *Principles of epidemiology.* Atlanta, GA: U.S. Department of Health and Human Services.

———. 1990. Summary of notifiable disease, United States 1989. *Morbity and Mortality Weekly Report* 38:1–59.

———. 1990. Update: Salmonella enteritidis infections and shell eggs—United States, 1990. *Morbidity and Mortality Weekly Report* 39:909–912.

Frazier, W. C., and D. C. Westhoff. 1978. *Food microbiology*, 3rd ed. New York: McGraw–Hill.

Marshall, P. G. 1988. How safe is your food? *Congressional Quarterly's Editorial Research Reports* 1:18.

Werner, S. 1992. Food poisoning. *Public health and preventive medicine*, 193–201, ed. J. Last and R. Wallace. Norwalk, CT: Appleton and Lange.

CHAPTER 11

Case Study of an Epidemic

Introduction

The investigation of what appears to be an epidemic is important from two aspects. First, it must result in a correct and definitive conclusion. Second, the assembled results must convince individuals with less technical knowledge of epidemiology that the findings are justified.

   The general rules that the investigator uses in presenting the results successfully are honesty, logicalness, and simplicity. The following steps give a sequence of tasks that will usually result in a correct conclusion when identifying an epidemic. The sequence will need to be modified as the events of the investigation are being done.

Outline of Procedure

   I. Establish the presence of an epidemic.
      A. Verify the diagnosis.
         1. Clinical findings. Review all clinical findings and, if needed, begin appropriate laboratory tests.
         2. Reliability. Establish that the laboratories, the physician, and other data sources are acceptable.
         3. Diagnostic methods. Question whether all the usual laboratory or clinical methods are needed. For some diseases no applicable laboratory tests exist. Other diseases can be verified only by laboratory findings. Can the required laboratory tests be performed by the average laboratory or is a highly specialized laboratory needed?
         4. Immediate reporting. Ask the health department to request an immediate reporting of all such cases that may not have been recognized or reported.
      B. Divide the cases into categories of definite, probable, or suspect.

C. Compare the disease incidence with "normal." Note the significance of the distinct departure from normal incidence or previous experience with the disease in question.

II. Establish the epidemic's parameters. The time, place, and persons related to the disease can be established by doing the following things.

A. Create a chronological distribution of the onset of cases according to days, weeks, or months. Some diseases' onset will have to be measured in hours.

B. Lay out the geographical distribution of the area affected. Use spot maps to determine the concentration in given areas.

C. Establish specific attack rates. With the available population data, codify the number of reported cases and deaths. Examine the data by sex, age, occupation, and location of residence to discern which groups were selected for attack.

D. Attempt to classify the preliminary epidemic data as to mode of transmission, as either common vehicle or propagated. The common vehicle cases can be subdivided as to whether they are "single exposure" (point of source) or "continued exposure." Divide the propagated cases into categories of "person-to-person spread," "anthropod vector," or "animal reservoir of infection."

Ascertain whether the epidemic's plotted curve is suggestive of a group of people being infected at or about the same time. Fix the probable time of the epidemic's occurrence based on the incubation period of the disease.

III. Formulate a tentative hypothesis of probable source.

IV. Create a plan of action. Decide how the sick will be cared for to facilitate minimization of the disease's spread. Decide how a detailed investigation of all cases or an unbiased sample of cases will be done. Establish how special collateral investigations can be conducted using specific laboratory facilities, engineering, and other expert consultations.

V. Analyze the data. As rapidly as case investigation data is assembled, compare the attack rate among the various pertinent groups. Identify, if possible, the universe (group) selected for attack and discover the common source or sources to which individuals were exposed.

A. Classify exposed individuals as to the following: exposure to specific potential vehicles; whether ill or not; and, if ill, clinical data and bacteriological findings to substantiate the diagnosis.

B. Investigate the source and method of any suspected food's preparation and preservation.

C. Perform collateral studies of environmental conditions, i.e., the sanitary status of the eating facilities, water, milk supply, and examination of food residues.

D. Demonstrate whether there are significant variations of incidence in contrasting population groups. From sample data in sections of the area (e.g., city wards or sanitary districts) and the population in question, calculate attack rates by race, sex, age, and occupational status.

For more detailed records, group cases according to sources of water supply, milk supply, ice cream supply, character of residence, and particular events or habits. Calculate the attack rates for each individual exposed and for those individuals not exposed to each vehicle; and the frequency of exposure to suspected vehicles, among those attacked and those not attacked.

E. Assemble the results of collateral investigations.

F. Search for human or animal sources of infection. Finally, test the various hypotheses the data seem to suggest, to ascertain which one is consistent with all the known facts. Further, seek out facts until an array is found that matches all deductions from one hypothesis and is inconsistent with all other hypotheses. Remember to base conclusions on all the pertinent evidence rather than relying on any single distribution or circumstance by itself.

Case Study: Bridgewater's Unusual Event

In the small town of Bridgewater a number of cases of a certain illness recently occurred. Neither the symptoms nor diagnosis of the illness will be given to you. From the epidemiological data provided, you will be able to characterize the epidemic by the variables of place, time, and person; develop a hypothesis about the disease involved, its source, and its mode of transmission; and establish the probable period of exposure to the source of the agent.

An investigation of Bridgewater's problems was initiated and revealed the following characteristics:

1. Among Bridgewater residents there were a total of thirty cases. This total represented more cases than had occurred in the past few years.

2. Case investigations were conducted and provided a set of data for each case. Included among the data were each case's age, address, sex, school and grade attended, or place of employment/occupation. Table 11.1 lists these selected case characteristics.

3. The milk consumed came from approved dairies but from various sources.

TABLE 11.1 Selected Characteristics of Cases in Bridgewater

No.	Case	Age	Sex	Onset	Address	Place Employed/Occupation or School and Grade
1.	R.D.	22	M	2/21/91	220 Main	Service station #1
2.	J.S.	5	F	2/22/91	318 Court	Bridgewater Elementary School
3.	R.B.	30	F	2/22/91	316 Main	Housewife
4.	S.S.	15	M	2/22/91	330 Court	Bridgewater High School
5.	R.J.	18	M	2/23/91	402 Oxford	Service station #2
6.	M.M.	33	F	2/23/91	315 Oxford	Bridgewater Elementary School (7)
7.	T.R.	8	F	2/24/91	230 Oxford	Bridgewater Elementary School (3)
8.	J.R.	6	M	2/25/91	230 Oxford	Bridgewater Elementary School (1)
9.	A.S.	27	F	2/26/91	230 Main	Bank
10.	H.A.	35	M	2/26/91	330 Main	Farm in country
11.	I.M.	34	F	2/27/91	422 Main	Housewife
12.	G.S.	9	F	2/27/91	318 Main	Parochial school
13.	C.M.	11	M	2/28/91	402 Court	Bridgewater Elementary School (6)
14.	K.C.	25	F	2/28/91	229 Court	Memorial Hospital (nurse's aide)
15.	J.E.	7	M	2/28/91	220 E. 3rd	Parochial school
16.	D.F.	14	F	3/2/91	230 E. 4th	Bridgewater Jr. High
17.	D.P.	12	M	3/2/91	401 Oxford	Bridgewater Elementary School (6)
18.	J.A.	10	F	3/3/91	115 E. 4th	Bridgewater Elementary School (5)
19.	D.H.	14	M	3/3/91	115 E. 4th	Bridgewater Jr. High
20.	J.V.	22	M	3/4/91	220 E. 4th	Unemployed
21.	D.T.	43	F	3/5/91	308 Oxford	Housewife
22.	V.K.	8	F	3/5/91	216 Court	Parochial school
23.	J.C.	11	M	3/5/91	116 E. 3rd	Bridgewater Jr. High
24.	G.A.	30	M	3/5/91	320 E. 4th	Hardware store
25.	L.C.	14	F	3/7/91	128 E. 3rd	Bridgewater Jr. High
26.	M.E.	10	F	3/7/91	210 E. 4th	Bridgewater Jr. High
27.	G.W.	11	M	3/9/91	230 E. 3rd	Bridgewater Jr. High
28.	B.R.	13	F	3/11/91	318 Main	Bridgewater High School
29.	C.H.	15	M	3/12/91	230 Court	Bridgewater High School
30.	B.E.	8	M	3/15/91	222 E. 3rd	Bridgewater Elementary School (3)

4. The four Bridgewater schools all have separate cafeterias and sources of food. There were no illnesses detected among students attending the Bridgewater schools who live outside of Bridgewater.

5. Bridgewater has a city water system, which provides the drinking water for Bridgewater residents.

6. All homes in Bridgewater are connected to the Bridgewater sewage system.

7. None of those individuals who were ill at the time of their first visit to Bridgewater had any visitors from outside of Bridgewater during the two months prior to this epidemic.

8. The brother of case number 21 and his family (himself, his wife, and four children) from a nearby state had visited her home on

TABLE 11.2 Population of Bridgewater by Age Group

Age Group	Number in Each Group
0–4	1,000
5–9	2,000
10–14	2,500
15–19	1,500
20+	7,000
Total	14,000

February 5 and 6. When case number 21 became ill, she learned that her brother and two of his children had become ill two days before coming to Bridgewater for their visit. Their symptoms were similar to those affecting case number 21.

Solving the Bridgewater Epidemic

Disease Surveillance

Using the eight characteristics just listed and Tables 11.1 and 11.2, what specific sources of information would you use in your search for additional epidemic-associated cases?

Characterizing the Epidemic

Prepare a table, graph, and chart which describe the epidemic by time, place, and person. Label neatly and legibly each with an appropriate title, adding labels and legends as needed for clarity. Round all calculations to one decimal place.

A. Time
1. Employ a histogram to construct an epidemic curve of Bridgewater's data.
B. Place
1. Create a spot map that indicates the location of each Bridgewater case by place of residence (Figure 11.1).
2. Construct a table to show the distribution of the cases based on their "place of employment/occupation or school and grade." Include your calculated percentage of the total number of cases in each age group.
C. Person
1. Prepare a table which describes the cases by sex and age group. Calculate and include the appropriate attack rates for each age group.

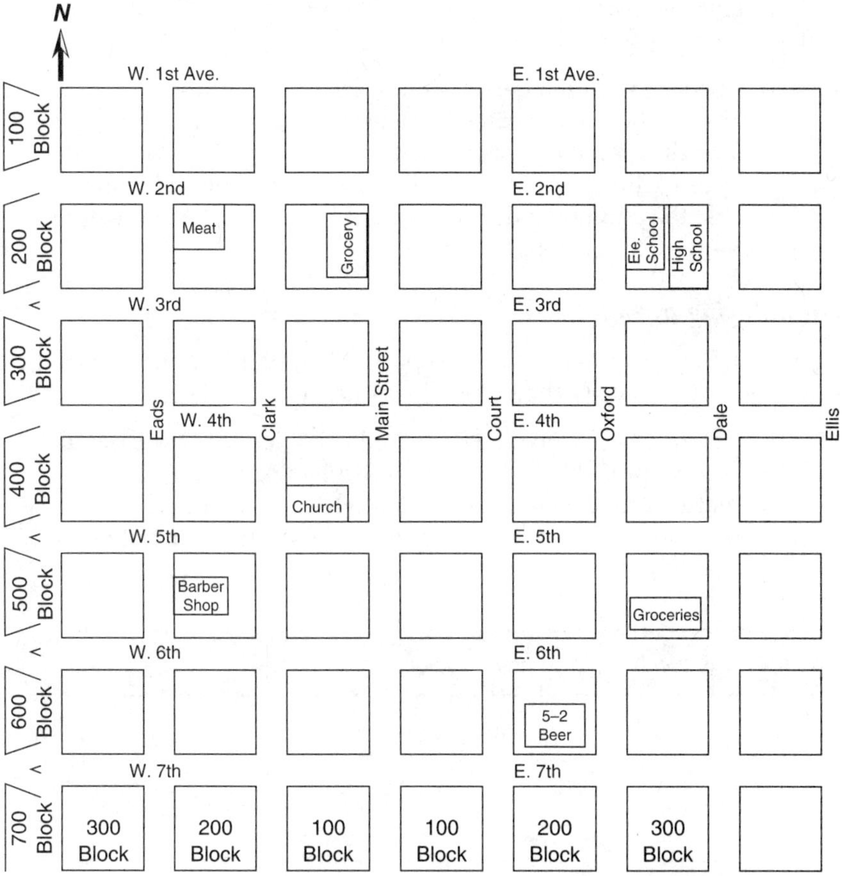

FIGURE 11.1
City of Bridgewater
Street Map.

NOTE: On East-West streets, even-numbered addresses are on the north side;
on North-South streets, even-numbered addresses are on the east side.

2. Calculate the ratio of the attack rate in the remaining
   Bridgewater population. In a single sentence explain the
   meaning of the ratio.
3. Calculate the mean and the median ages for each sex
   category. Be sure to use a work sheet to share your
   calculations.
4. Calculate a ratio, comparing the mean ages by sex
   category.

Analyzing the Data

Now begin to analyze the data of Bridgewater's epidemic employing
your histogram of the epidemic curve; spot map of the case's locations;

table of employment/occupation and school/grade; table of cases' sex and age group; and ratio of mean age by sex.

    A. Prepare a written description of the occurrence and distribution of the cases from each of the tables.
    B. List the limitations of the analyses that were imposed by the type of information you were provided for this epidemic.
    C. List the additional disease surveillance activities you would suggest at this point.

Formulating a Hypothesis

Now, based on your analysis of the epidemic, prepare a written hypothesis in which you specify the following information:

    A. The disease involved. Using Table 11.3, identify the disease that is most probably involved with Bridgewater.
    B. Nature of the source. Figure out whether the source is a common source or a propagated source or a combination of both types.

TABLE 11.3 Incubation Periods of Selected Diseases

Disease	Incubation Period		Maximum Expected Duration of a Point-Source Epidemic*
	Average	Minimum/Maximum	
Amebic dysentery	21–28 days	5 days to several months	8 days +
Anthrax	2–5 days	2–7 days	6 days
Brucellosis	5–21 days	5 days to several months	17 days
Diphtheria	2–5 days	2–5 days +	4 days +
Food poisoning:			
Staphylococcal	2–4 hours	1–6 hours	6 hours
Clostridium			
perfringens	10–12 hours	8–22 hours	15 hours
Hepatitis A	28–30 days	15–50 days	36 days
Leptospirosis	10 days	4–19 days	16 days
Measles	10 days	8–13 days	6 days
Poliomyelitis	7–12 days	3–21 days	19 days
Rabies	14–42 days	10–180 days	171 days
Rocky Mountain			
Spotted fever	—	3–10 days	8 days
Salmonellosis	12–24 hours	6–48 hours	43 hours
Shigellosis	4 days	1–7 days	7 days
Syphilis	3 weeks	10 days to 10 weeks	61 days
Trichinosis	9 days	2–28 days	27 days
Typhoid fever	14 days	7–21 days	15 days

*Assuming simultaneous exposure of a large number of susceptibles (based on the minimum incubation periods).

C. Mode of transmission. Determine how the disease was transmitted—by direct contact, vehicleborne, or some other method.
D. Period of time. Determine the time frame during which the cases were most likely to have been exposed.

Testing the Hypothesis

You have started with your "best assumption" as to just what happened in Bridgewater. Next you must briefly describe for each part of your hypothesis the steps that would be taken to confirm that hypothesis.

A. What specific methods should you use to confirm your hypothesis?
B. Which specific information would you collect to confirm your hypothesis?

When you have completed your case study, consult the back of this text for the suggested solutions. With the key, you will be able to score each completed section of the case study with your written response.

Note the material used in this case study was provided by the Epidemiology Program Office, U.S. Department of Health and Human Services, Centers for Disease Control and Prevention, Atlanta, Georgia.

CHAPTER 12

Chronic Disease Epidemiology

Introduction

Chronic diseases are often referred to as chronic illnesses, noncommunicable diseases, and/or degenerative diseases. In general, they are characterized by uncertain etiology, multiple risk factors, a long latency period, a prolonged course of illness, a noncontagious origin, some type of functional impairment or disability, and a rarely achieved curability. Often, however, the characteristics of chronic and acute diseases overlap, such as with the case of AIDS, tuberculosis, mental illness, drug addition, and occupational health disorders. Thus, any definition may need to be flexible to account for a wide range of diverse disease processes (Brownson, Remington, and Davis 1993).

Epidemiologists have identified several individual **risk factors** that are related to many of the major chronic diseases (Table 12.1). It is evident from Table 12.1 that the control of a single risk factor, such as obesity, may reduce the risk of several chronic diseases. In addition to the risk factors listed in the table, there are also many genetic and physiological factors that may place one at greater risk of some chronic diseases.

Chronic Disease Methodology

The presence of a single known necessary cause, as in the case of measles, syphilis, and salmonella, greatly assists epidemiologists in shaping their research and intervention strategies. In comparison, chronic diseases lack such unifying causal agents in that the disease process is generally protracted and complex, having multiple causes. Thus, intervention strategies require a multifaceted approach.

Brownson and his colleagues (1993) suggest that in order to understand the methodological principles in chronic disease epidemiology, one needs to examine them from the perspective of a particular goal. One might, for example, consider the role of a public health officer who is seeking to describe the patterns of a particular disease occurrence, identify opportunities for control, and recommend a strategy for public health

TABLE 12.1 Interrelationships between Various Chronic Diseases and Modifiable Risk Factors, United States

	Cardiovascular Disease	Cancer	Chronic Lung Diseases	Diabetes
Tobacco use	+	+	+	
Alcohol use	?	+		
High cholesterol	+			
High blood pressure	+			
Diet	+	+	?	?
Physical inactivity	+	+		+
Obesity	+	+		+
Stress	?	?		
Environmental tobacco smoke	?	+	+	
Occupation		+	+	
Pollution		+	+	
Low socioeconomic status	+	+	+	+

	Cirrhosis	Musculoskeletal Diseases	Neurological Disorders
Tobacco use		+	?
Alcohol use	+	+	+
High cholesterol			
High blood pressure			
Diet		+	?
Physical inactivity		+	
Obesity		+	+
Stress			
Environmental tobacco smoke			
Occupation	?	+	?
Pollution			+
Low socioeconomic status	+	+	

Source: From Brownson, R., P. Remington, and J. Davis. 1993. Chronic disease epidemiology and control. Washington, D.C.: American Public Health Association.

Note: + = established risk factor; ? = possible risk factor.

programs. From this perspective, an epidemiologist might ask the following questions with respect to heart disease:

1. How much heart disease is occurring?
2. How does the occurrence of heart disease vary within this population?
3. How does the burden of heart disease in this area compare with other areas?

4. What types of investigations are done to study the etiology and control of heart disease?
5. How can we evaluate whether the study results are valid?
6. How can we assess whether the associations between potential etiological factors and heart disease are causal?
7. How much of the morbidity and mortality from heart disease might be prevented from interventions?

The following sections will examine these questions in depth with respect to one chronic disease—lung cancer. In this way, we will be able to apply these epidemiological questions to a serious public health problem.

Occurrence of Lung Cancer in a Population

In order to investigate this factor, an epidemiologist needs to quantify the magnitude of the occurrence of lung cancer in a geographical region. To quantify the problem, the researcher might consider using measures such as incidence, cumulative incidence, and prevalence (see Chapter 6).

Incidence rates are typically employed to describe the number of new cases that develop in a year in a specified population. For example, if 132 people developed lung cancer in 1991 in a city with a population of 150,000, the incidence rate for that city would be 88 per 100,000 population. Comparing this to the total U.S. population, the incidence rate for lung cancer in men was 80 per 100,000 in 1991, whereas for women the corresponding incidence rate was 41 (American Cancer Society 1994).

The risk of developing a disease over a defined time period is referred to as the *cumulative incidence*. In this regard, the risks of dying from lung cancer are twenty-two times higher for male smokers and twelve times higher for female smokers than for those people who have never smoked.

Prevalence rates are influenced by the incidence (new cases) and persistence of the disease and by rapid recovery or rapid death. These rates are generally less valuable for identifying etiological factors. In lung cancer, the five-year survival rate for all stages of cancer is only 13 percent (American Cancer Society 1994). For many chronic diseases, such as diabetes and coronary heart disease, mortality rates are calculated because incidence data are not available.

Variance of Occurrence in a Population

Data from the Applied Research Branch of the National Cancer Institute (Table 12.2) shows the risk of being diagnosed with the most common cancers over certain age intervals for each sex. Note that the measures do not take into account individual risk factors, such as smoking, or exposure to carcinogenic substances, such as asbestos, radiation, radon, or sidestream smoke. Thus, the risk for a nonsmoking woman developing lung cancer during her lifetime is much lower than 5.02 percent, and it is much higher for a smoker.

TABLE 12.2 Percentage of Population (Probability) Developing Invasive Cancers at Certain Ages

		Birth to 39	40 to 59	60 to 79	Ever (Birth to Death)
All sites	Male	1.68 (1 in 60)	7.51 (1 in 13)	32.27 (1 in 3)	42.52 (1 in 2)
	Female	1.91 (1 in 52)	9.29 (1 in 11)	23.06 (1 in 4)	38.88 (1 in 3)
Breast	Female	0.45 (1 in 222)	3.78 (1 in 26)	6.78 (1 in 15)	12.20 (1 in 8)
Colon & rectum	Male	0.06 (1 in 1,667)	0.91 (1 in 110)	4.45 (1 in 22)	6.12 (1 in 16)
	Female	0.05 (1 in 2,000)	0.73 (1 in 137)	3.34 (1 in 30)	5.96 (1 in 17)
Prostate	Male	Less than 1 in 10,000	0.78 (1 in 128)	10.71 (1 in 9)	13.05 (1 in 8)
Lung	Male	0.04 (1 in 2,500)	1.60 (1 in 63)	6.69 (1 in 15)	8.43 (1 in 12)
	Female	0.03 (1 in 3,333)	1.07 (1 in 93)	3.49 (1 in 29)	5.02 (1 in 20)

Source: From Applied Research Branch, National Cancer Institute. 1993.

Note: This chart shows the risks of being diagnosed with the most common cancers over certain age intervals. These risks are calculated for persons free of the specified cancer at the beginning of the age interval. Risk estimates do not assume all persons live to the end of the age interval or to any fixed age. Risk estimates are presented to give an approximate measure of the burden of cancer to society. Measures are based on population level rates and do not take into account individual behaviors and risk factors. For example, lung cancer is rare among nonsmokers or persons not heavily exposed to environmental tobacco smoke, so the risk for a nonsmoking man getting lung cancer in his lifetime is much lower than 8.4%, and it is much higher for a smoker. It is clear that the risk of developing cancer increases with age. For prostate cancer, the risk before age 60 is very low, but between age 60 and 80, 1 in 9 men will be diagnosed with prostate cancer.

TABLE 12.3 Smoking Related Rate Ratio (Relative Risk) and Rate Difference Estimates for Coronary Heart Disease and Lung Cancer among Women, United States, 1982–1986.

| | Mortality Rate | | Rate | |
Disease	Smokers (a)	Nonsmokers	Ratio (a/b)	Difference (a–b)
Lung cancer	131	11	11.9	120
Coronary heart disease	275	153	1.8	122

Source: From Office on Smoking and Health. 1989. *Reducing the health consequences of smoking: 27 years of progress*. A report of the Surgeon General. Washington, D.C.: U.S. Department of Health and Human Services.

As shown in Table 12.3, the relative risk (ratio of the cumulative incidence or risk in two groups) due to smoking among women is much greater for lung cancer than for coronary heart disease. Notice, however, that the rate difference for heart disease for the four-year period is greater than the rate difference for lung cancer. This is due to the fact that the death rate for heart disease is much greater than the death rate for lung cancer in women.

Comparison of Lung Cancer in a Specific Area with Other Areas

Local, state, and federal health agencies publish incidence rates for different types of cancers, including lung cancer. This enables health officials to compare their local incidence or mortality rates with other geographical areas.

Epidemiologists can also examine the variance of lung cancer among other regions, states, and nations. For example, the death rate in the United States for lung cancer in males is 57.1 per 100,000 population, as compared to males in Sweden, where it is 23.4. The corresponding figures for females are 24.7 and 9.9, respectively (American Cancer Society 1994).

One should be cautious, however, in making comparisons among different geographical areas because one area may have a higher proportion of aged people, in which cancer rates are apt to be higher. In order to make an adequate comparison, one needs to adjust each rate to a standard population by combining age-specific rates into an age-adjusted rate. For example, the lung cancer rates for the United States and Sweden have been age-adjusted to the World Health Organization world standard population. Another problem that may arise when comparing small regions is that the incidence or mortality rate may be low for a given year. In order to obtain a better perspective, rates should be compared over several years.

Types of Investigations Used to Study Lung Cancer

The major types of observational studies that have been extensively used in lung cancer epidemiology are the prospective (cohort) study and the retrospective (case-control) study (see Chapter 8). Table 12.4 summarizes the strengths and limitations of prospective and case-control studies for review purposes.

There is another type of study, or disease-control strategy, in which an educational program or screening program is systematically offered to a population and the effect on health is measured. This is the **quasi-experimental intervention study**. In this type of study, the major objective is to determine how effective an intervention program was, e.g., in preventing smoking from occurring or in getting smokers to stop smoking. Unfortunately, such studies require comparison groups, which are often lacking, or sometimes the comparison group is not sufficiently appropriate (Brownson, Remington, and Davis 1993).

Quasi-experimental intervention study–a type of study design that is used when randomization of subjects is not feasible, usually in cases where intact groups are available, such as schools, institutions, etc.

A 1989 Surgeon General's Report (U.S. Department of Health, Education, and Welfare 1989) summarizes the three major types of smoking prevention approaches: (1) media-based prevention programs and resources; (2) smoking prevention as part of a multicomponent school health education curriculum; and (3) psychosocial approaches of social influence and generic life skills curricula.

Media-based prevention efforts by themselves have not been shown to prevent youth from smoking. However, these approaches may serve as effective complements to school-based curriculum approaches (Flay 1986).

TABLE 12.4 Summary of Strengths and Weaknesses of Prospective (Cohort) and Retrospective (Case-Control) Studies

Study Type	Strengths	Weaknesses
Prospective (cohort)	Valuable when exposure is rare Can study multiple effects of a single exposure Provides the opportunity to measure risk factors before disease occurs Can measure incidence rates as well as relative risk Minimizes bias	Generally not efficient for studying rare diseases Can be expensive and time consuming Requires a large number of subjects Validity of results may be affected by subject attrition Requires lengthy follow-up period
Retrospective (case-control)	Quick and inexpensive Useful for studying diseases with protracted latent periods Useful for rare diseases May examine multiple etiological factors for a single disease	Presents possible bias in measuring risk factors after disease has occurred Prone to bias in subject recall Possible bias in selecting comparison group Temporal relationship between exposure and disease may be difficult to establish

A number of curriculum-based programs have been found to delay the onset of initial smoking experimentation and the development of regular smoking practices, but the desired long-term effects have not generally been achieved. Many variables may intervene, such as the problems inherent in teacher training, teacher variation in implementation, and adherence to the prescribed lessons, as well as cultural socioeconomic differences within the school groups (Best et al. 1989; Flay 1985; Stone and Mulhall 1993). Other factors, such as the counter influence of advertising, peer pressure, and lack of well-defined school policies, may also have a confounding effect.

Community trials, such as the Stanford Three Community Study, have shown some promising results. The Stanford study involved three small communities of approximately 20,000 residents. Individuals in each community were nonrandomly assigned to control, media only, and media and face-to-face study groups. The researchers found that the prevalence of smoking decreased the most in the intensive intervention group (media and face-to-face) and that 32 percent of those who stopped smoking sustained their cessation after the study (Meyer et al. 1980).

The North Coast Study in Australia, using a similar approach, found that their intensive approach group showed a 6 to 15 percent smoking decrease whereas the control group had a small decrease of 1 to 5 percent in smoking prevalence. In this study the intensive media program also included a physician intervention program in stress management and physical fitness (Egger et al. 1983).

TABLE 12.5 Suggestions for Avoiding Bias in Epidemiological Studies

A. Basics for a sampling plan
1. Each individual in the population must have an opportunity or a known probability for inclusion in the sample(s). Groups selected must be exactly alike in all respects except for the factor under study.
2. Basic rules
   a. The population sampled must be well-defined and include all persons in the population.
   b. Each person must have a known probability of inclusion in the sample.
   c. The sampling plan must be sharply defined and strictly followed.
3. Confirm comparability of cases and comparison subjects. Adequately check samples for characteristics other than those used for selecting the study population.
4. Special considerations in retrospective and prospective studies
   a. Internal comparisons should be used between case and comparison groups to establish equivalence.
   b. The methods of selecting the comparison group should permit control of confounding variables.
   c. The term *control* implies a situation that an investigator seldom has in the study of human disease and health. *Comparison group* is a more suitable term.

B. Nonrespondents and dropouts
1. Avoid nonrespondents and dropouts when possible, and obtain data from several independent sets of records or by attempting additional follow-up efforts. Substitutes cannot overcome the loss of data from nonrespondents or dropouts.
2. Investigate a subsample of, or have another basis for estimating, the known characteristics of nonrespondents or dropouts. If you can demonstrate that the known characteristics of respondents and nonrespondents are similar, you can have more confidence that their nonresponse has not introduced a bias. These measures are only a partial replacement for nonresponse and cannot prove that the data are not biased.

C. Self-selection
1. In general, volunteers are usually better educated, more strongly motivated, and more consistent in following instructions. They may be more likely to show a beneficial effect from treatment. Therefore, results from a study using volunteers may not be replicable in the general population.
2. The use of volunteers may be unavoidable when medical procedures or measurements are to be performed or evaluated, especially when multiple examinations are required over a long period of time.
3. Identify the characteristics of the volunteers and attempt to estimate the effect of using subjects who are self-selected.
4. The randomization of volunteers to treatment may be a necessary and useful research tool in many situations.
5. Be aware that the effect of some types of self-selection may tend to either diminish or increase with time.

D. Subjectivity
1. In experimental studies, subjectivity may be avoided by *double-blind* techniques.
2. Subjectivity can be avoided or minimized by the use of objective tests, independent observers unaware of background information, or certain types of written records that do not rely on subjective opinions for interpretation.
3. Extreme efforts are often necessary to establish standard and uniform procedures to assure precise data collection.

TABLE 12.5 Suggestions for Avoiding Bias in Epidemiological Studies—cont'd

E. Interobserver variation
1. Use the same observers for case and comparison groups.
2. Record and adjust for interobserver differences.
3. Subsample independently or interchange observers.
4. As a last resort, discard data from incompetent observers.

F. Misclassification
1. Minimize errors by using objective criteria whenever possible.
2. When dealing with historical information, minimize errors by training interviewers and data collectors, using precise definitions, and exercising scrupulous care.

Source: Adapted from White, C. 1982. In Roht, L., B. Selwyn, A. Holquin, and B. Christensen, *Principles of epidemiology: A self-teaching guide.* New York: Academic Press, 419–420.

Despite certain limitations, such as lack of a comparison group, quasi-experimental studies such as community-wide and school programs have shown that low cost intervention studies can have an impact on the population's health (Farquhar et al. 1990). Additional methods used to reduce smoking include smoking cessation classes; government and private sector measures, such as banning smoking in buildings, airplanes, and restaurants; increasing insurance rates for smokers; workplace restrictions; limiting advertising; increasing federal, state, and local taxes on cigarette purchases; and no-smoking policies in schools.

Evaluating the Validity of Study Results

Brownson and his colleagues (1993) state that "the most useful framework in which to consider potential errors in epidemiological studies is to ask why the calculated measure of association, such as relative risk, may not accurately reflect the causal impact of exposure in disease." In a study on lung cancer, for example, if one obtains a relative risk (an odds ratio) of 12.0, why are we not confident that introducing exposure to the variable of smoking will increase the risk of developing lung cancer twelve-fold? The reason is that several different types of bias may affect the relative risk and present distortions in the findings. The information in Table 12.5 gives some examples of the types of bias that may exert an impact on the validity of study results.

Bias often cannot be totally eliminated, but a good researcher should attempt to anticipate potential sources. All epidemiological studies contain certain limitations, which may be inherent in the study design, availability and/or accuracy of data, and so forth. Because of this, researchers devote a considerable amount of effort to eliminate or control those aspects of their research that are likely to result in bias.

Assessing Causality

Certain criteria have evolved to enable researchers to judge when the association of a factor (such as smoking) may be considered a causal association, which may in part explain the etiology of a disease (such as lung cancer) and/or account for its pattern. These criteria are as follows:

1. The strength of the association should be high, as reflected by a high relative risk.
2. The time sequence should appear to be logical in that exposure preceded the disease onset.
3. The association should be specific for the disease, i.e., the exposure causes one rather than many diseases. When only a few causal factors can produce a disease, there will be a stronger association between that disease and the separate factors than if there are numerous causal factors.
4. The association should be consistent in that it is observed among diverse populations and circumstances, making a particular bias unlikely to explain a series of such observations.
5. The association should agree with known biological facts or theories. The evidence that has accumulated from other studies should suggest that the agent is biologically capable of influencing the disease and hence offers a plausible explanation.

In this section we will discuss the epidemiological criteria for establishing whether or not an observed association plays a causal role in the etiology of lung cancer. The data are from the Surgeon General's Report on Smoking and Health (1979). The report provides epidemiological data derived from retrospective, prospective, and cross-sectional studies. Remember that retrospective studies assist in establishing the presence of an association between variables and provide a measure of the strength of the association by estimating relative risks. Prospective studies measure the incidence rate (new cases) of a disease, which follows exposure to variables suspected of having an association with the disease. Cross-sectional studies determine the prevalence of various diseases.

In the past thirty years, more than fifty retrospective studies on the relationship between cigarette smoking and lung cancer have been published. All of the studies have shown an association between lung cancer and smoking. Thus, the weight to be attached to the consistency of the findings in the retrospective studies is enhanced when one considers that these studies all differed in their methods and sample sizes.

In addition, there have been at least nine major prospective studies that have examined the relationship between cigarette smoking and mortality from various causes. The results from eight of these studies—those involving cigarette smoking and lung cancer—are presented in Table 12.6. Note that the lowest mortality ratios are experienced by female smokers, whereas the highest mortality ratios for males vary from 3.8 to 14.0. In combining the data from the largest studies, one can deduce that cigarette smokers, on the average, are ten times more likely to develop lung cancer than nonsmokers.

These studies, taken together, illustrate a consistency of observation given widely dispersed and varying study methods. Also, the relative risks resulting from the different methods are consistently and greatly in excess of 2.0.

TABLE 12.6 Lung Cancer Mortality Ratios—Prospective Studies

Population	Size	Number of Deaths	Nonsmokers	Cigarette Smokers
British doctors	34,000 males	441	1.00	14.0
Swedish study	27,000 males	55	1.00	8.2
	28,000 females	8	1.00	4.5
Japanese study	122,000 males	590	1.00	3.76
	143,000 females	148	1.00	2.03
A.C.S. 25-state study	440,000 males	1,159	1.00	9.20
	562,000 females	183	1.00	2.20
U.S. veterans	239,000 males	1,256	1.00	12.14
Canadian veterans	78,000 males	331	1.00	14.2
A.C.S. 9-state study	188,000 males	448	1.00	10.73
California males in 9 occupations	68,000 males	368	1.00	7.61

Source: From U.S. Department of Health, Education, and Welfare. 1979. Smoking and health: A report of the Surgeon General. Washington, D.C.: Government Printing Office.

The data in Table 12.7, which provide death rates from lung cancer, are taken from the classic study on smoking and lung cancer by Doll and Hill (1950). The data illustrate another aspect of the strength of the association, as demonstrated by the dose response to smoking. As the dose increases, the relative risk of death increases from 8.1 to 32.4 for heavy smokers.

Mortality ratios for all cancers are about twice as high in smokers as in nonsmokers. Thus, most cigarette smokers are about twice as likely as nonsmokers to die of cancer. The highest mortality ratio is for lung cancer, followed by cancer of the larynx, oral cavity, esophagus, urinary bladder, and pancreas.

The mortality ratio for all of the cardiovascular diseases is about 1.6, with the mortality ratio for coronary heart disease in several studies ranging from 1.3 to 2.03. We know that there are several important risk factors for the development of coronary heart disease, including cigarette smoking, hypertension, and high blood cholesterol. None, however, appears to be more important than cigarette smoking.

The criteria we have discussed illustrate the specificity of the association between an agent and a disease. It appears that smoking plays a role in many diseases but that its greatest impact is on lung cancer. Thus, cigarette smoking is more likely to play a direct and causal role in lung cancer than in other diseases.

TABLE 12.7 Death Rates and Relative Risk from Lung Cancer by Daily Cigarette Consumption (1951–1961)

Cigarettes per Day	Death Rates per 1000 per Year	Relative Risk
0	0.07	—
1–14	0.57	8.1
15–24	1.39	19.9
25+	2.27	32.4

Source: From U.S. Department of Health, Education, and Welfare, 1979. Smoking and health: A report of the Surgeon General, Washington, D.C.: Government Printing Office.

Table 12.8 gives the data for lung cancer mortality ratios for males according to the age when they began smoking. What does this information illustrate? It provides indirect evidence to show the temporal relationship between exposure to the agent and the onset of the disease. As we mentioned earlier, exposure to the agent must precede the onset of the disease.

Clinical, experimental, pathological, and epidemiological studies of humans and animals have clearly demonstrated that cigarette smoking produces measurable lung damage. These findings collectively illustrate the criterion of coherence, in that a plausible mechanism is suggested by the overwhelming available evidence.

Preventing Lung Cancer by Intervention

The reduced prevalence of smoking suggests that millions of smokers have stopped smoking and a substantial proportion of them have remained abstinent for many years. While most of these ex-smokers have stopped without the help of formal programs and clinical interventions, a variety of formal programs have developed to assist people who want to quit but need help doing so. In addition, the social climate has created an unfavorable tolerance toward smokers, with strict controls being placed on smoking in most public and private facilities; higher federal, state, and city cigarette taxes; and more emphasis on prevention programs.

For persons who stop cigarette smoking, the lung cancer mortality decrease is gradual, and after ten years the risk may still be 30 to 50 percent of the risk for continuing smoking. However, the lung cancer mortality decrease is related to several factors, such as dose, duration, type of cigarette, and depth of inhalation, as well as the number of years since cessation of smoking (Felding 1992). Calculating the attributable and relative risk of smoking may be particularly useful in evaluating the potential benefits of intervention (see Chapter 8).

TABLE 12.8 Lung Cancer Mortality Ratios for Males, by Age Began Smoking, from Selected Prospective Studies

	Age Began Smoking in Years	Mortality Ratio
A.C.S. 25- state study	Nonsmoker	1.00
	25+	4.08
	20–24	10.08
	15–19	19.69
	Under 15	16.77
Japanese study	Nonsmoker	1.00
	25+	2.87
	20–24	3.85
	Under 20	4.44
U.S. veterans	Nonsmoker	1.00
	25+	5.20
	20–24	9.50
	15–19	14.40
	Under 15	18.70

Source: From U.S. Department of Health, Education, and Welfare. 1979. Smoking and health: A report of the Surgeon General. Washington, D.C.: Government Printing Office.

Summary

This chapter explains some of the methodological issues in chronic disease epidemiology by focusing on lung cancer to illustrate basic epidemiological concepts. Methodological principles as well as different types of observational studies are discussed and their strengths and weaknesses are explored. The importance of attempting to be cognizant of research limitations and bias are stressed.

Criteria for assessing causality are illustrated to determine if an observed association between cigarette smoking and lung cancer can provide a sufficient basis to ascertain causality. Epidemiological data gleamed from retrospective, prospective and cross-sectional studies are used to strengthen the role of cigarette smoking in the etiology of lung cancer. Lastly, the prevention of lung cancer by employing intervention techniques is discussed.

Discussion Questions

1. Define chronic disease. How does it differ from acute disease?
2. Briefly discuss the major questions a public health officer might ask regarding lung cancer in his or her community.

3. Present several examples of how bias may be avoided or minimized in epidemiological studies.
4. What are the advantages and disadvantages of prospective and retrospective studies?
5. Cite and explain an example of a community trial.
6. Describe the criteria for assessing causality.

References

American Cancer Society. 1994. *Cancer Facts and Figures.* Atlanta, GA: ACS.

Best, J., et al. 1989. Preventing cigarette smoking among school children. *American Review of Public Health* 9:161–201.

Brownson, R., P. Remington, and J. Davis. 1993. *Chronic disease epidemiology and control.* Washington, D.C.: American Public Health Association.

Doll, R., and A. Hill. 1950. Smoking and carcinoma of the lung. *British Medical Journal* 1:739–748.

Egger, G., et al. 1983. Result of a large scale media antismoking campaign in Australia, North Coast "Quit for Life" Programme. *British Medical Journal* 286:1125–1128.

Farquhar, J., et al. 1990. Community education for cardiovascular health. *Lancet* 8023:1192–1195.

Fielding, J., 1992. Smoking: Health effects and control. In J. Last and R. Wallace, eds. *Public health and preventive medicine*, Norwalk, CT: Appleton and Lange.

Flay, B. 1986. Mass media linkages with school-based programs for drug abuse prevention. *Journal of School Health* 56:402–406.

Flay, B. 1985. What we know about the social influences approach to smoking prevention: Review and recommendations. In Bell, C., and R. Battjes, eds. *Prevention research: Deterring drug abuse among children and adolescents*, No. (ADM) 85–1334:67–112. Washington, D.C.: U.S. Department of Health and Human Services.

Meyer, A., et al. 1980. Skills training in a cardiovascular health education campaign. *Journal of Consulting Clinical Psychology* 48:129–142.

Stone, D., and P. Mulhall. 1993. Project drug free. Paper presented at the SOPHE Annual Conference, San Francisco, October 1993.

U.S. Department of Health and Human Services. 1989. Reducing the health consequences of smoking: 25 years of progress. A report of the Surgeon General. No. 89–8411. Washington, D.C.: Government Printing Office.

U.S. Department of Health, Education and Welfare. 1979. Smoking and health. A report of the Surgeon General. Washington, D.C.: Government Printing Office.

CHAPTER 13

Epidemiology and Health Policy

Introduction

Epidemiology has played a significant role in the development of national health policy. The fundamental activities of epidemiology—observation, enumeration, hypothesizing, and identifying relationships—have formed the cornerstone upon which much of health policy making has developed. From the time of Shattuck and others, the epidemiological method has generated much of the evidence upon which national health policy decisions have been made.

In this chapter we will examine the role epidemiological information plays in developing health policy. We will approach this overview by examining some specific instances in which epidemiological data have influenced health policy. It is important to note that policy formulation is not based solely on an objective interpretation of data, which identifies a cause and suggests a potential means of intervention in health problems. In reality, additional factors must be considered, including the effects of economic, scientific, ethical, and political feasibility.

Questions ranging from "What to do with the Broadstreet pump?" to "How to best deal with the AIDS epidemic?" have been answered, in part, through epidemiological reasoning. But there are many policy dimensions in these questions as well. This is clearly illustrated in the current debate over the barring of HIV+ individuals from entry into the United States. An epidemiological rationale, which suggests that such individuals pose no threat to the public health of Americans, has not deterred to date a policy of nonadmittance, which is based in part on the potential economic impact such individuals might have on the U.S. health-care system.

Let us examine several instances in which epidemiological reasoning and information have played a key role in policy formulation.

The Swine Flu Immunization Program

Perhaps no single modern event better illustrates the role of epidemiology in the formulation of health policy than the swine flu immunization program. This national immunization program was instituted as a result of events that occurred primarily during 1976 and 1977. From a historical perspective, the immunization campaign was partly a reaction to the fear that a pandemic of a strain of flu dubbed the "swine flu," which had occurred prior to the 1920s, was about to be repeated. The initial cause for concern was the death of a soldier at Fort Dix, New Jersey, in February of 1976. His death, which had been attributed to swine flu, was a major cause for concern as were five additional confirmed cases and eight other probable cases occurring at Fort Dix. The prospect that these events might indeed be signaling the advent of a new potential pandemic of the suspected flu necessitated a swift examination and evaluation of the epidemiology of swine flu. Moreover, the events necessitated an evaluation that would hopefully lead to a sound policy aimed at effectively dealing with the potential threat of a national and possibly worldwide epidemic.

The subsequent events, decisions, and policies have become the subject of praise in some circles and significant criticism in others. The decision to begin a national swine flu immunization campaign was made in March of 1976. It was put forth to the American people on the basis of the recommendation of a blue-ribbon committee of experts. The committee concluded that such immunizations were needed in terms of their effectiveness in primary prevention and were appropriate in terms of their margin of safety. Architects of the immunization program justified the need for the massive immunization efforts based on a "better safe than sorry rationale." While few were critical of the approach in terms of its appropriateness regarding a pending epidemic, others were highly skeptical of the conclusions that were drawn from the available epidemiological evidence.

Even prior to the onset of the immunization program, a major sign of controversy and disagreement involved the potential efficacy and safety of the immunization program itself. This was painfully illustrated in the initial refusal of companies carrying liability insurance for the vaccine's manufacturers to underwrite the production and sale of the vaccine. This refusal necessitated the intervention of the Federal government, which became, in essence, the liability insurer for the vaccine. Following the introduction of the swine flu immunization program, the death of three elderly inoculees signaled a new wave of concern and criticism. The increasing difficulty of promoting a national immunization campaign for a disease that still was not in evidence beyond the Fort Dix cases was further complicated by another disturbing series of events.

The Centers for Disease Control identified a somewhat rare condition known as Guillain-Barre syndrome in a number of swine flu inoculees. The condition has the potential for causing permanent paralysis and even death in some cases. The occurrences of this condition became the final bit of evidence that subsequently resulted in the termination of the immunization program. Detractors of the national immunization policy speculated that the program was ill-advised and faulty for a number of reasons (Wecht 1978):

1. The epidemiological evidence often cited for the formulation of the program did not justify the conclusion of a pending epidemic.
2. The epidemiological investigations into the potential effectiveness and safety of the vaccine were tainted by a prior judgment in favor of a national immunization campaign.
3. The significance of the epidemiological information in terms of formulating the policy that initiated the immunization program was both clouded and to some extent motivated by political necessity. The issue of how a successful immunization policy might influence the pending presidential elections may have been given more weight than epidemiological evidence in the decision to proceed with such a program.
4. Once begun, the immunization program was difficult to terminate without losing face despite mounting evidence indicating that termination of the program was necessary.

In summary, critics believe that the epidemiological evidence was given less than adequate consideration. They also find that political concerns may have unduly influenced the immunization policy, which led to the often maligned national program. On the other hand, those who defend the program suggest that the epidemiological evidence justified a vigorous response based on the understanding of what an epidemic of the swine flu might do to an unprotected public. Policy analysts stress that the events leading to the swine flu immunization program indicate a need for additional appropriate mechanisms to help translate epidemiological information into effective health policies (Fielding 1978).

Injury Prevention and Control

While the concept of "having an accident" is a common, if undesirable, notion to most individuals, the means and methods of studying accidents is less well known. Indeed, the paradigms for the study of accident prevention and control have undergone a continuing development based on the use of epidemiological methods. The very term *accident* has fallen out of favor among injury experts due to the increasing understanding of the causes and outcomes of accidents. This increased understanding is the result of examining injury prevention and control in the light of the epidemiological triad—host, agent, and environment.

Studying "accidents" in this manner allows epidemiologists to examine the three elements of the triad at various points in time. In its most basic form, examining the elements prior to an event (e.g., a car crash or fall), during an event, and following an event supplies investigators with significant information. This information may often be useful in understanding the causes of the event and possibly averting similar occurrences. Data that are gathered to identify what transpired during an event such as a crash or fall may provide vital information on potential means of minimizing future injuries. Examining post-event information can also provide us with the knowledge of how best to provide acute and rehabilitative care for injuries. It is this epidemiological approach to injury prevention and control that is responsible for the current maxim, "injuries are no accident." In other words, the popular concept of an accident as an unpredictable and random event is untrue. While the plaintive cry of "I'm sorry, it was an accident!" may mean that the individual did not intend for the event to happen, it should not be interpreted as meaning that the accident was not predictable and preventable.

In the area of injury prevention and control, a significant contribution to policy development has been in the most fundamental activity of epidemiology, the enumeration of injuries. The information that is gathered citing the number and nature of injuries in America has provided new insights into the significance and scope of this public health problem.

Epidemiological data suggest that, in terms of lost years of productive life, two health problems have emerged as the major contributors. The first, communicable diseases, has received considerable attention in terms of the development of public health policy measures. Improvements related to policies in housing, sanitation, potable water supplies, working conditions, and school immunizations have significantly diminished the impact of infectious diseases on our population.

The second health problem, which has now emerged as the leading cause of lost years of productive life, is that of injury. Epidemiological data presented in a landmark study, *Injury in America, 1985*, depicts the extent to which injury is a major factor in the death and disability of Americans. As the fourth leading cause of death, injury is responsible for approximately 150,000 deaths per year. Within specific age groups, the figures are particularly alarming. Injury causes almost half the deaths of children aged 1–4, more than half the deaths of children aged 5–14, and nearly four–fifths of the deaths of persons aged 15–24. The two major chronic diseases, in terms of mortality, do not surpass injuries as a cause of total deaths until age 45. Interestingly, injuries are the leading cause of physician contacts, surpassing diseases, which might be expected to have accounted for the bulk of doctor-patient interactions. Injury is also the leading cause of both short- and long-term disability.

A subsequent study, *Cost of injury in the United States, a report to Congress, 1989*, notes that the economic toll of injury in terms of productivity loss far exceeds the three other causes of death that rank above it. Policies that govern priorities—in terms of the resources directed to the prevention and control of specific health problems—appear to be inconsistent with the allocations one would expect based on epidemiological evidence.

If we compare the resources directed to injury prevention with those directed to the two major chronic disease areas, cancer and heart disease, vast disparities are apparent. The congressional report just cited documents that injury research expenditures are significantly less than in others areas. The report states that ". . . injury research expenditures by all federal agencies amounted to $160 million in 1987, about one tenth of the National Cancer Institute expenditures and one sixth of the expenditures of the National Heart, Lung and Blood Institutes."

Policy recommendations to raise expenditures aimed at the prevention and control of injuries have increased markedly in recent years. Of particular concern has been the disturbing trend of increased death and disability due to intentional injuries such as murders, assaults, or suicides *(Promoting Health/Preventing Disease, Objectives for the Year 2000).* While recommendations to increase spending are based on an understanding of the epidemiology of injuries as we have discussed, policy changes still must overcome the misunderstood nature of "accidents" as chance occurrences that are, by definition, not preventable.

Healthy People 2000—Priorities

The use of epidemiological data to influence policy is a historical fact, as evidenced in our earlier discussions of the Shattuck report (see Chapter 2). Within the past twenty years several national policy documents, including *New Perspectives on the Health of Canadians* (Lalonde 1972) in Canada, and *Healthy People* (U.S. Department of Health and Human Services 1979) have used epidemiological arguments that national health policies are in need of redirection. That redirection can be generalized as the need for policies that emphasize increased "self responsibility" for health. This suggestion is based on an understanding of the role that individual life-styles play in contributing to a person's health status. This policy emphasis is evident in the *Promoting Health and Preventing Disease, Objectives for the Nation, 1990* and *Healthy People 2000.*

The challenges and goals set forth in *Healthy People 2000* are divided into three major areas: health promotion, health protection, and preventive services.

Epidemiological data are used to present baseline status figures and accompanying objectives for the nation. The report paints a profile of the health of the American people, documents progress in health status for the past ten years, and sets specific goals and objectives for the year 2000. These goals and objectives are intended to direct the health improvement strategies of the 1990s. The achievement of three broad goals are identified as the purpose of *Healthy People 2000:*

1. To increase the span of healthy life for Americans
2. To reduce health disparities among Americans
3. To achieve access to preventive services for all Americans

The final series of objectives within the document target strategies for enhancing our epidemiological ability to monitor health and disease trends. These objectives deal with the area of surveillance. They address the "systematic collection, analysis, interpretation, dissemination and use of health information." These objectives underscore the fact that the effectiveness of any health policy is in part a function of the validity and timeliness of the epidemiological data upon which it is based.

Summary

This chapter examined the role that epidemiology plays in the development of health policy. While epidemiological data provide the basis for analytical reasoning, often other factors such as economics, politics and medical ethics enter into the development of policy formulation. Specific events such as the development of the swine influenza immunization program, injury prevention and control, and the establishment of health priorities are examined from this perspective.

The swine influenza immunization program was presented as an example of how epidemiological evidence was manipulated by various factions to influence immunization policy. Also, the broad area of injury control was presented to illustrate how policy development and implementation can become intertwined with priorities regarding resource allocation and the need for expanding public health programs.

Finally, the major goals of increased life span, reduction of health disparities, and access to preventive health services for all Americans are presented to emphasize that effective health policy implementation demands valid and timely epidemiological data.

Discussion Questions

1. Describe the role that politics, economics and medical ethics played in health policy with respect to the swine influenza immunization program.
2. Present the major evidence presented by detractors of the national swine influenza immunization program.
3. Describe the magnitude of the injury problem in the United States.
4. Why do you think injury control programs are insufficiently funded in comparison to heart disease and cancer?
5. Describe the major goals set forth in *Healthy People 2000*. Do you think such goals are reasonable? Why or why not?
6. What role does epidemiology play in the development of health policy? What other factors besides epidemiological data enter into health policy decisions?

References

Fielding, J. 1978. Managing public health risks: The swine flu immunization program revisited. *American Journal of Law and Medicine* 4:35–43.

Healthy people 2000. U. S. Department of Health and Human Services. 1990. DHHS publication No. (PHS) 91–50212. Washington, D.C.: Government Printing Office.

Lalonde, M. 1974. *New perspectives on the health of Canadians.* Ottawa, Canada: Ministry of National Health and Welfare.

National Research Council and the Institute of Medicine. 1985. *Injury in America, a continuing public health problem.* Washington, D.C.: National Academy Press.

Promoting health/preventing disease, objectives for the year 2000. Washington: U.S. Department of Health and Human Services, 1989 (draft).

Rice, D., E. MacKenzie et al. 1989. *Cost of injury in the United States, a report to congress, 1989.* Institute for Health and Aging, University of California and The Injury Prevention Center, Baltimore, MD: Johns Hopkins University.

U. S. Department of Health, Education and Welfare. 1979. *Healthy people: The surgeon general's report on health promotion and disease prevention.* Washington, D.C.: Government Printing Office.

Wecht, C. 1978. The swine flu immunization program: Scientific venture or political folly? *American Journal of Law and Medicine* 77:426–445.

CHAPTER 14

Epidemiology
and the Future

Introduction

As we have seen in previous chapters, the role of epidemiology within society has continued to evolve, and disease surveillance continues to be recognized as a major function of epidemiologists. Given the potential of technology to deal with some of the causes of morbidity and mortality, and the successful conquests of numerous communicable diseases, we might conclude that the role of epidemiology would be lessening in importance. However, the practice of epidemiology is assuming greater significance in several interrelated areas. Let us examine a few of the areas in which epidemiology may have increasing influence in future years.

Epidemiology and Social Behavior

Traditionally, epidemiology has been applied to the prevention and control of communicable and chronic diseases. Increasingly, though, the methods of epidemiology are being applied to the study of additional societal problems outside the domain of traditional public health. The study of behavior-related causes of morbidity and mortality has expanded the scope of traditional epidemiology beyond disease causation. If current trends continue, epidemiologists will study such public health concerns as the distribution and determinants of intentional violence and individual risk analysis. The practice of epidemiology is becoming increasingly important to health professionals in environmental, occupational, and educational areas (Lane 1987).

The increasing disability and mortality that are related to assaults, murders, and suicides indicates that intentional injury is a significant societal problem. Researchers examining the problem of intentional violence predict an even greater problem in the future (Rosenberg 1991). Public health practitioners have urged that this problem needs to be analyzed in a manner similar to other classic public health problems. They suggest that epidemiological methods are necessary if we are to accurately define the nature of the causes of intentional violence and develop effective interventions. Marzuk, Tardiff, and Hirsch (1992) suggest the development of standardized operational definitions of violence in its many forms, and coordinated surveillance networks as a necessary foundation for prevention efforts. Future efforts to understand and curb intentional violence will also require a scientific understanding of the social context in which individuals live. The need for social epidemiologists to work cooperatively with other interested parties to better understand the precursors of intentional violence is paramount (Earls 1991). The principles that have formerly been applied to disease investigation will need to be applied to other social problems. The complex interrelationships between social risk factors will place increasing demands on epidemiologists to develop new analytical techniques and investigative methodologies. The application of epidemiological methods to social problems such as intentional violence indicate the evolving training and competencies that will be required for the interdisciplinary work of the future.

Epidemiology and Developing Countries

The role of epidemiology in improving the health status of developing countries will continue to be a significant one. The incorporation of epidemiological data into systematic health planning can greatly enhance the potential cost benefit and cost effectiveness of health services. This application of epidemiological study may be particularly critical in developing countries where comprehensive population data bases are in need of development (Okoli 1990). As stressed by Morrow and Lansang (1991), epidemiological study directly related to the needs of people in developing countries is not only essential in formulating effective health planning, but also is necessary in addressing the issue of equity of services. The need for interdisciplinary collaboration is essential. Such an approach will require the development of regional and national training centers for the preparation of skilled personnel. The demand for increasingly sophisticated epidemiological surveillance in developing countries will have a major impact on the need for trained professionals (Frerichs 1991).

In addition to disease surveillance, developing countries also are generating the kinds of problems often associated with more advanced countries. As pointed out by Levy et al. (1992) epidemiological research is necessary in the areas of environmental and occupational health as well as communicable and chronic disease surveillance. Rates of occupational and environmental illness and injuries are often higher in developing countries. Unfortunately, epidemiological research capabilities and resources in these countries are often limited.

Although the attention of epidemiologists has, in the past, focused on the study of communicable diseases in developing nations, it is apparent that the scope of epidemiological research will expand in the future. Intentional and unintentional injuries are another area of increasing concern in developing countries. The epidemiological study of these events will aid in planning an effective approach to tragedies that may occur (Shears 1991). Tragedies such as the famines in Ethiopia and Somalia have focused the world's concern on food supply and the citizens of developing nations. Epidemiologists stress that increased study must occur on the nutritional problems of Third World residents (Brown and Solomons 1991).

The nature of the population dynamics of developing countries may at times be characterized as transient and nonstationary. These characteristics necessitate a variety of specialized epidemiological techniques—incorporating population growth rate, transience of the population, and population density—in order to develop sound public health policies (Tuljapurkar 1991).

Epidemiology will continue to play an important role in the evolving health status of developing nations. Specialized epidemiological research investigating such diverse areas as child psychiatry (Nikapota 1991), acute respiratory infections (Berman 1991), HIV (Broekmans 1991) and maternal morbidity (Liskin 1992) exemplify the future range of challenges.

Epidemiology and History

In considering the future role of epidemiology in society, it is interesting to note the linkage between history and the future. Epidemiology has provided several lessons to us concerning the relationships between society, disease, and health status. As outlined by Vutela and Tuomilehto (1992), the evolution of the social environment of a society is a major determinant of the health and disease trends within that society. Historically, epidemiology has traced how social development has significantly contributed to the decrease in traditional public health problems and the emergence of new ones. The time lag between changes in social trends and disease patterns makes the meaningful application of epidemiological data in health planning challenging. Epidemiology can play a crucial role, for example, in addressing the evolving health problems of Eastern Europe, as they are related to social developments, just as epidemiology assisted in addressing the health problems of earlier days (Vutela and Tuomilehto 1992). Several authors have pointed out the historical lessons that epidemiology has taught in relation to how we might deal with present and future diseases of concern. Ampel (1991) notes that while medical science has made great strides in overcoming infectious disease, several epidemics of previously unrecognized diseases have occurred within the past fifteen years. These epidemics have included Lyme disease, Legionnaire's disease, toxic shock syndrome, and AIDS. A historical review of epidemics of disease shows some parallels with current diseases of concern. In an analysis of four past epidemics (the plague of Athens, the Black Death, syphilis, and influenza) Ampel noted similarities and differences between past and present occurrences of disease. Epidemics seem to appear in cycles and abate over time due to changes in the infecting pathogen or changes in the host. New infectious agents, which are produced by the mutation of a pathogen to a virulent form, may be introduced into a nonimmune population via environmental and behavioral factors. This fact suggests that epidemiologists need to be students of history as well as prognosticators of future disease trends.

Fox (1989) similarly suggests that the successful epidemiologists of the future will need to be students of the lessons of epidemiological history. In particular, he suggests that the lessons of epidemiology offer some guidance for understanding the social and policy responses to the AIDS epidemic. Society's reactions to past epidemics have included an initial underestimation of the severity of the epidemic; the rise of fear and anxiety; and flight, denial, and scapegoating. These reactions closely parallel the early reactions to the AIDS epidemic.

Epidemiologists of the future may also have to deal with viruses and bacteria that emerge in new forms or reemerge in old forms in new populations due to life-style factors. Thus, epidemics connect the future with the past, offering lessons for guarding the health of future generations (Krause 1994).

Emerging Infectious Diseases

As defined by the CDCP, emerging infectious diseases "refer to diseases of infectious origin whose incidence in humans has either increased within the past two decades or threatens to increase in the near future" (Centers for Disease Control 1994). As we can see in Table 14.1, many factors may interact to contribute to disease emergence, such as the mutation or evolution of existing organisms, the spread of existing diseases to new populations, or the appearance of previously unrecognized infections in persons living or working in areas undergoing ecological changes (e.g., deforestation or reforestation). In the latter, there may be increased human exposure to insects, animals, or environmental sources that may serve as reservoirs of new or unusual infectious agents (Krause 1981; Morse and Schluederberg 1990; Epstein 1992). Also infectious diseases may reappear because of the development of antimicrobial resistance in existing agents (e.g., malaria, gonorrhea, pneumococci) or because of a breakdown in public health measures used for previously controlled infections (e.g., cholera, tuberculosis, pertussis) (Centers for Disease Control 1994). Furthermore, infectious agents may be causing diseases previously considered noninfectious. For example, helicobacter pylori has shown a strong association with peptic ulcers and gastritis (Blaser 1991); sexually transmitted human papillomavirus with cervical cancer (Reeves et al. 1989); and the hepatitis virus with chronic liver disease and cirrhosis (Alter 1992). In addition, epidemiological studies have implicated chlamydia infections with infertility and coronary artery disease (Kou et al. 1993),

Categories	Specific Examples
Societal events	Economic impoverishment; war or civil conflict; population growth and migration; urban decay
Health care	New medical devices; organ or tissue transplantation; drugs causing immunosuppression; widespread use of antibiotics
Food production	Globalization of food supplies; changes in food processing, packaging, and preparation
Human behavior	Sexual behavior; drug use; travel; diet; outdoor recreation; use of day-care facilities
Environmental changes	Deforestation/reforestation; changes in water ecosystems; flood/drought; famine; global warming
Public health infrastructure	Curtailment or reduction of prevention programs; inadequate communicable disease surveillance; lack of trained personnel (e.g., epidemiologists, laboratory scientists, and vector and rodent control specialists)
Microbial adaption and change	Changes in virulence and toxin production; development of drug resistance; microbes as cofactors in chronic diseases

Source: From Centers for Disease Control. 1994. Addressing emerging infectious disease threats: A prevention strategy for the United States. *Morbidity and Mortality Weekly Report* 43 (RR–5).

Giardiasis–an infection caused by a protozoan that displays a person-to-person transmission by hand-to-mouth transfer of cysts from the feces of an infected individual, especially in institutions and day-care centers. Humans serve as the principal reservoir, although beavers and other wild and domestic animals may also be a source.

Cryptosporidiosis–a parasitic infection caused by a coccidian protozoan that is fecally excreted and present in polluted water as a highly resistant, relatively small oocyst. Humans, cattle, and other domestic animals serve as a reservoir for the organism.

and rodentborne hantaviruses may play a role in hypertensive renal disease (Glass et al. 1993).

Consequently, the threat of emerging infections appears to be increasing as concomitant changes in society, technology, and the environment occur along with the evolution and spread of pathogens. In the past several decades, the U.S. public health system has been challenged by newly identified pathogens and syndromes, such as Legionnaire's disease, Lyme disease, toxic shock syndrome, the hepatitis C virus, and hantavirus pulmonary syndrome. Moreover, the incidence of many diseases thought to be controlled (i.e., cholera, dengue, yellow fever, and tuberculosis) has increased in many areas or spread to new regions in the world. Also, due to the widespread use and misuse of antimicrobial drugs, their effectiveness in treating common bacterial infections is being diminished, resulting in prolonged illness, higher mortality rates, and correspondingly higher health costs (Centers for Disease Control 1994).

Newly emerging infections are particularly serious in persons with suppressed immunity, such as those infected with HIV and those receiving immunosuppressive therapy for cancer or organ transplantation, as well as the elderly, persons in institutions such as hospitals and nursing homes, the homeless, migrant workers, and those with inadequate access to health care.

In the United States, more than eleven million children are attending day-care facilities and are at substantially increased risk for enteric infections such as hepatitis A, acute respiratory illnesses, middle ear infections, **giardiasis** and **cryptosporidiosis**. And those children who become infected may infect other members of a household (Thacker et al. 1992).

In 1993, the intestinal parasite cryptosporidium, transmitted by contaminated public water supplies, caused the largest recognized outbreak of waterborne disease ever recorded in the United States. This emerging infection caused an estimated 403,000 people to become sick with prolonged diarrhea. In this same year, hamburgers contaminated with escherichia coli served at a fast food chain caused a multistate outbreak of bloody diarrhea and serious kidney disease, resulting in the deaths of at least four children. Both of these pathogens were first recognized as important emerging microbes in the early 1980s but have not received adequate public health attention (Centers for Disease Control 1994).

Travel and commerce have aided in the worldwide spread of pathogens such as HIV/AIDS and influenza, as well as in the reemergence of cholera as a global health threat. These examples underscore the fact that emerging infections can affect large groups of people in geographically widespread areas of the world.

The surveillance of infectious diseases in the United States depends on voluntary cooperation between the CDCP and state and local health departments, which in turn rely on reporting by health-care professionals dedicated to infectious disease surveillance. Unfortunately, in many states there is an inadequate number of professional positions devoted to infectious disease surveillance as well as inadequate funding (Centers for Disease Control 1994).

Epidemiology and Public Policy

A traditional role of the epidemiologist is one of an impartial observer, a scientist-recorder of information who provides valid information which can be utilized in policy formulation. As we saw in Chapter 13, however, epidemiologists have become involved in formulating policy and, in some cases, accused of shaping epidemiological data to "fit" a predetermined policy outcome (Colby and Cook 1991). To be sure, epidemiology has been recognized as the foundation for sound health policy. In commenting on future needs in epidemiology, Vuori (1992) suggests that it must be the basis for achieving the World Health Organization goal of "health for all." He suggests that epidemiological inquiry is best able to assist in identifying health problems, setting achievable and measurable goals, and providing a basis for outcome evaluation.

The future of epidemiology will be a challenging one. The areas discussed within this chapter suggest that not only will the challenges be technical, in terms of developing increasingly sophisticated methodologies, but will also involve interaction with other professionals. These future interactions will involve challenges in the area of professional ethics as well. The ethical implications for the use of epidemiological data in public policy development are substantial. Gordis (1991) has pointed out that as the nature of the practice of epidemiology changes, new ethical and professional issues must be addressed. As the role of epidemiologists continues to evolve, health professionals and the general public as well will gain an increasing understanding and appreciation for epidemiology.

Summary

This chapter focuses on issues in which epidemiology may play an ever expanding role in the twenty-first century. Such areas as social behavior, improving the health status of newly developing countries, emerging infectious diseases, and public policy are examined with respect to future concerns and issues relevant to the field of epidemiology.

It is anticipated that epidemiology will assume a more active role in the areas of violence reduction and social risk factors. The need to more fully understand the precursors of intentional violence is underscored as well as the need to develop new competencies for effective interdisciplinary cooperation with other allied health practitioners.

The application of epidemiological methods in formulating effective health planning in newly developing countries is discussed. Research in the areas of child psychiatry, acute respiratory infections, and maternal morbidity as well as population growth typify the range of new challenges to epidemiology.

Similarities of certain diseases such as the Black Death and syphilis with AIDS are discussed. Such parallels are important to understand with respect to societal attitudes and public reactions to health programs.

Newly emerging infectious diseases threaten to increase in future decades due to the mutation and evolution of existing organisms. Such factors as economic impoverishment, urban decay, the widespread uses of antibiotics, the expansion of day-care facilities, changes in our ecosystems, new medical devices, and immunosuppressive drug therapies are examples of specific factors contributing to the threat of emerging diseases.

Lastly, this chapter addresses the need for epidemiologists to develop more sophisticated methodologies as well as calling for a need to be concerned with ethical issues.

Discussion Questions

1. Discuss how epidemiology is increasing its scope in studying new public health concerns in the area of social behavior.
2. What role can epidemiology play in the evolving health problems of developing nations?
3. Discuss the major factors contributing to the emergence of infectious diseases.
4. Why are newly emerging diseases a threat to public health both in the United States and other countries?
5. Why do epidemiologists need to be students of history as well as prognosticators of future disease trends?

References

Alter, M., et al. 1992. The natural history of community acquired hepatitis C in the United States. *New England Journal of Medicine* 321:1899–1905.

Ampel, N. 1991. Plagues—what's past is present: Thoughts on the origin and history of new infectious diseases. *Reviews of Infectious Diseases* 13 (4):658–665.

Berman, S. 1991. Epidemiology of acute respiratory infections in children of developing countries. *Reviews of Infectious Diseases* 13 (Supplement 6):454–462.

Blaser, M., et al. 1991. Association of infection due to helicobacter pylori with specific upper gastrointestinal pathology. *Reviews of Infectious Diseases* 13:704–708.

Broekmans, J. 1991 Tuberculosis and HIV infection in developing countries. *Tropical and Geographical Medicine* 43 (3):13–21.

Brown, K., and N. Solomons. 1991. Nutritional problems of developing countries. *Infectious Disease Clinics of North America.* 5 (2):297–327.

Centers for Disease Control. 1994. Addressing emerging infectious disease threats: A prevention strategy for the United States. *Morbidity and Mortality Weekly Report* 43 (RR5).

Colby, D., and T. Cook. 1991. Epidemics and agendas: The politics of nightly news coverage of AIDS. *Journal of Health Policy, Politics, and Law* 16 (2):215–249.

Earls, F. 1991. Not fear nor quarantine, but science: Preparation for a decade of research to advance knowledge about causes and control of violence in youths. *Journal of Adolescent Health* 12 (8):619–629.

Epstein, P. 1992. Commentary: Pestilence and poverty— historical transitions and the great pandemics. *American Journal of Preventive Medicine* 8:263–265.

Fox, D. 1989. The history of responses to epidemic disease in the United States since the eighteenth century. *Mount Sinai Journal of Medicine* 56 (3):223–229.

Frerichs, R. 1991. Epidemiologic surveillance in developing countries. *Annual Review of Public Health* 12:257–280.

Glass, G., et al. 1993. Infection with a ratborne hantavirus in U.S. residents is consistently associated with hypertensive renal disease. *Journal of Infectious Diseases* 167:614–620.

Gordis, L. 1991. Ethical and professional issues in the changing practice of epidemiology. *Journal of Clinical Epidemiology* 44 (Supplement 1):9–13.

Kou, C., et al. 1993. Demonstration of chlamydiapneumoniae in atherosclerotic lesions of coronary arteries. *Journal of Infectious Diseases* 167:841–849.

Krause, R. 1981. The restless tide: The persistent challenge of the microbial world. Washington, D.C.: National Foundation for Infectious Diseases.

Krause, R. 1994. The origin of plagues: Old and new. *Science* 257 (5073):1073–1078.

Lane, J. C. 1987. Social epidemiology: Directions for the future. *Journal of Community Health* 12 (2):130–138.

Levy, B., et al. 1992. Ongoing research in occupational health and environmental epidemiology in developing countries. *Archives of Environmental Health* 47(3): 231–235.

Liskin, L. 1992. Maternal morbidity in developing countries. *International Journal of Gynecology and Obstetrics* 37 (2):77–87.

Marzuk, P., K. Tardiff, and C. Hirsch. 1992. The epidemiology of murder-suicide. *Journal of the American Medical Association* 267 (23):3194–3195.

Morrow, R., and M. Lansang. 1991. The role of clinical epidemiology in establishing essential national health research capabilities in developing countries. *Infectious Disease Clinics of North America* 5 (2):395–404.

Morse, S., and A. Schluederberg. 1990. Emerging viruses: The evolution of viruses and viral diseases. *Journal of Infectious Diseases* 162:1–7.

Nikapota, A. 1991. Child psychiatry in developing countries. *British Journal of Psychiatry* 158:743–751.

Okoli, J. C. 1990. Epidemiology, the root of prevention of disease and pointer to better provision of health services. *West African Journal of Medicine* 9 (4):330–334.

Reeves, W., et al. 1989. Epidemiology of genital papillomaviruses and cervical cancer. *Reviews of Infectious Diseases* 11:426–439.

Rosenberg, M. 1991. Violence as a public health problem. Lecture: Birmingham, AL: UAB Injury Prevention Research Center.

Shears, P. 1991. Epidemiology and infection in famine and disasters. *Epidemiology and Infection* 107 (2):241–251.

Thacker, S., et al. 1992. Infectious diseases and injuries in child day care: Opportunities for healthier children. *Journal of the American Medical Association* 268:1720–1726.

Tuljapurkar, S. 1991. Disease in changing populations: Growth and disequilibrium. *Theoretical Population Biology* 40 (3):322–353.

Vuori, H. 1992. Epidemiology and health for all. The role of epidemiology in health policy. *Social and Preventive Medicine* 37 (2):45–49.

Vutela, A., and J. Tuomilehto. 1992. Changes in disease patterns and related social trends. *Reviews of Infectious Diseases* 166:14–20.

Case Study of an Epidemic: Bridgewater's Unusual Event

Scoring Key

This scoring key is included to assist you in determining your ability to characterize the epidemic described in chapter 11 by the variables of time, place, and person. In addition, it should enable you to assess your development of appropriate hypotheses concerning (1) the disease involved, (2) the source, (3) the mode of transmission, and (4) the probable period of exposure to the source of the agent.

The exercise should be scored in two parts. Part I has a range of 0 to 69 points. A suggested score is as follows:

$$70–78 = A$$
$$61–69 = B$$
$$53–60 = C$$
$$45–52 = D$$
$$\text{Below } 44 = E$$

Part II focuses on your ability to properly analyze and draw appropriate conclusions from the data presented in Part I. An outline of suggested considerations is included to assist you in determining how well you were able to conduct this important analysis. It is suggested that you grade this part on a letter scale (A to E) according to your success in incorporating the major concepts into your responses.

Part I (69 Points)

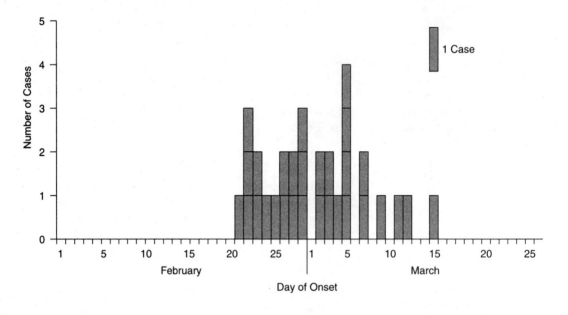

Error in cases	Points discounted
1	0
2–3	1
4–5	2
6–7	3
8 or more	4

2. Place 18
  a) Spot map of block of residence...................................6
    (1) Title. Is your title correct? 1
        (Distribution of epidemic-associated) cases of an
        (unknown) disease by block of residence,
        Bridgewater (USA), February (21)–March (15), 1991
    (2) Legend. Is the legend correct? 1
        Dot (spot)—1 case
    (3) Distribution of cases by block.........................4

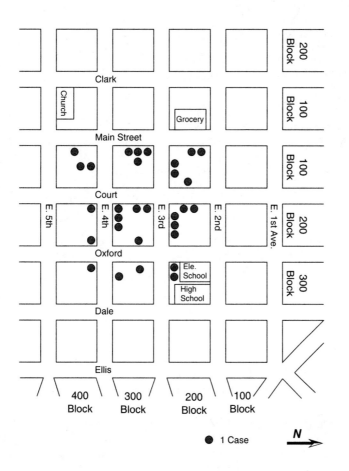

Error in cases	Points discounted
1	0
2–3	1
4–5	2
6–7	3
8 or more	4

    b) Table—Place employed/occupation or school.......21

        (1) Title. Is your title correct? 1
              (Distribution of epidemic-associated) cases of an (unknown) disease and percent of the total (cases by place employed/occupation), Bridgewater (USA), February (21)–March (15), 1991

Place Employed or School	Number of Cases	Percent
Bridgewater Elementary School	8	26.7
Bridgewater Jr. High School	6	20.0
Bridgewater High School	3	10.0
Parochial school	3	10.0
Housewife	3	10.0
Service station #1	1	3.3
Service station #2	1	3.3
Bank	1	3.3
Farm	1	3.3
Hospital	1	3.3
Hardware store	1	3.3
Unemployed	1	3.3
Total	30	99.8

        (2) Column or row omissions 9

	Points discounted
Case column	3
Percent column	3
Total row	3

        (3) Labels 4
             (*a*) Column...3
                  i) Place employed/occupation 1
                ii) Number of cases 1
                iii) Percent (of total)/% (of total) ..1
             (*b*) Row (total) 1
        (4) Categories of place employed/occupation or school 3
             (*a*) Minimum of 10 categories....................1
             (*b*) Each school should be listed separately (grade distributions may be shown and are acceptable, but total cases and percent should be shown for each school)..1

(c) Categories should be listed in descending order
     of frequency 1
(5) Numerical entries (cases/percentages) 4

Number inaccurate	Points discounted
1	0
2–3	1
4–5	2
6 or more	3
Percentages not rounded properly	1

C. Person ....C=20
  1. Table: Sex and age group 13
    a) Title. Is your title correct? 1
    (Distribution of epidemic-associated) cases of an
    (unknown) disease by age group, sex, and attack rates*
    (per 1,000 population) by age group, Bridgewater (USA),
    February (21)–March (15), 1991

| Age Group (Years) | Population | Number of Cases | | | Attack Rates |
		Male	Female	Total	
0–4	1,000	0	0	0	0.0
5–9	2,000	3	4	7	3.5
10–14	2,500	5	5	10	4.0
15–19	1,500	3	0	3	2.0
20+	7,000	4	6	10	1.4
Total	14,000	15	15	30	2.1

*Attack rates per 1,000 population.

    b) Column/row omissions

Column/row	Points discounted
Population	2
Male cases	2
Female cases	2
Total cases	2
Attack rates	2
Total row	2

    c) Labels. Are they correct? 6
      (1) Column 4
        (a) Age group (years) 1
        (b) Population...1
        (c) Number of cases—male, female,
          total 1
        (d) Attack rates..1
      (2) Row...2

    (*a*) Age groups.......................................1
    (*b*) Total...1
d) Numerical entries (population, cases, attack
    rates)..6

Inaccurate entries	Points discounted
1–2	1
3–4	2
5–6	3
7–8	4
9 or more	5
Attack rates not rounded correctly	1

2. Comparison of attack rates by age.......................2
  a) Ratio 1
  Ratio of attack rate in 10–14 year olds to that of the
  remaining population:
  Attack rate in 10–14 year olds = 4.0 cases/1,000
  population
  Attack rate in remaining population

$$= \frac{(30-10)}{14,000-2,500} \times 1,000$$
$$= \frac{20}{11,500} \times 1,000$$
$$= 1.7 \text{ cases}/1,000 \text{ population}$$
$$\text{Ratio} = 4.0 : 1.7$$
$$= 2.4 : 1.0$$

  b) Interpretation..1
  The attack rate (risk of acquiring illness) among 10–14
  year olds was 2.4 times greater than the attack rate (risk
  of acquiring illness) among the remaining population.
  Alternately: the number of cases per 1,000 population
  among the 10–14 year olds was 2.4 times greater than
  the number of cases per 1,000 population among the
  remaining population.

3. Calculation of the mean and median ages of the cases by
  sex...4
  a) Mean ages..2
    (1) Male mean age..................................1

$$= \frac{237}{15} = 15.8 \text{ years}$$

    (2) Female mean age...............................1

$$= \frac{283}{15} = 18.9 \text{ years}$$

b) Median ages 2
      (1) Male median age = 14.0 years 1
      (2) Female median age = 14.0 years 1
4. Comparison of the mean ages by sex 1
  a) Preferred answer
    Female mean age:male mean age

$$18.9:15.8$$
$$1.2:1.0$$

(The mean age of female cases was 1.2 times greater than the mean age of male cases)

  b) Acceptable answer
    Male mean age:female mean age

$$15.8:18.9$$
$$0.8:1.0$$

(The mean age of male cases was 8/10 or 80 percent that of the mean age of female cases)

5. Mean and median ages of the cases by sex
  a) Cases in males

←**Either**→

Age in Years	Cumulated Ages	Age in Years	No. Cases	$f_i x_i$	Σf_i	$\Sigma f_i x_i$
6	6	6	1	6	1	6
7	13	7	1	7	2	13
8	21	8	1	8	3	21
11	32	11	3	33	6	54
11	43	12	1	12	7	66
11	54	14	1	14	8	80
12	66	15	2	30	10	110
14	80	18	1	18	11	128
15	95	22	2	44	13	172
15	110	30	1	30	14	202
18	128	35	1	35	15	237
22	150					
22	172					
30	202					
35	237					

(1) Mean: total male cases = 15
    $\Sigma f_i x_i$ and Σx_i (summary of ages) = 237

$$\text{Mean} = \frac{237}{15} = 15.8 \ (15.80)$$

Mean age of male cases = 15.8 years

Case Study of an Epidemic   **185**

(2) Median:

$$\text{Intermediate point of distribution} = \frac{15+1}{2} = \frac{16}{2} = 8$$

The eighth observation falls in the interval = 14.0 years
Median age of male cases = 14.0 years

b) Cases in females

(1) Mean: total female cases = 15

$\Sigma f_i x_i$ and Σx_i (summary of ages) = 283

$$\text{Mean} = \frac{283}{15} = 18.9 \ (18.86)$$

Mean age of female cases = 18.9 years

←**Either**→

Age in Years	Cumulated Ages	Age in Years	No. Cases	$f_i x_i$	Σf_i	$\Sigma f_i x_i$
5	5	5	1	5	1	5
8	13	8	2	16	3	21
8	21	9	1	9	4	30
9	30	10	2	20	6	50
10	40	13	1	13	7	63
10	50	14	2	28	9	91
13	63	25	1	25	10	116
14	77	27	1	27	11	143
14	91	30	1	30	12	173
25	116	33	1	33	13	206
27	143	34	1	34	14	240
30	173	43	1	43	15	283
33	206					
34	240					
43	283					

(2) Median:

$$\text{Intermediate point of distribution} = \frac{15+1}{2} = \frac{16}{2} = 8$$

The eighth observation falls in interval = 14.0 years
Median age of female cases = 14.0 years

Answers

Preferred—Females:Males
18.9:15.8
1.2:1.0 (1.19:1.0)
(The mean age of female cases was 1.2 times greater than the mean age of male cases)
Acceptable—Males:Females
15.8:18.9
0.8:1.0 (0.83:1.0)
(The mean age of male cases was 8/10 that of the mean age of female cases)

Part II: Analysis and Conclusions

A. Time (histogram by day of onset)
  1. Duration of the epidemic
     a) February 21–March 15
     b) 23-day interval
  2. Peak (mode) occurred on March 5 (4 cases)
  3. Midpoint of the distribution (median date of onset) was March 1
  4. Period of exposure
     a) February 5 or 6 most likely
     b) Average of 28–30 days from median date of onset (January 28–February 1)
     c) Minimum incubation period (15 days) from first case and maximum incubation period (50 days) from last case (January 24–February 6)
  5. Incubation periods based on exposure on February 5 or 6
     a) Bridgewater cases—15–38 days
     b) Case #21 and relatives
        (1) Case #21 = 27–28 days
        (2) Relatives = 24–25 days
  6. Conclusion: Common-source exposure on February 5 or 6 to hepatitis A
  7. Limitations
     a) Diagnosis of cases lacking
     b) Temporal distribution of similar cases that have occurred in earlier periods are unavailable
B. Place
  1. Spot map
     a) All cases reside in a 9 square block area
        Alternatives
        (1) All cases in an area of 9 blocks bounded by Main, E. 2nd, Dale, and E. 5th
        (2) Two-thirds or 66.7 percent of the cases occurred in 4 square blocks
     b) Comparison of risk by block of residence cannot be accomplished without population data
     c) Conclusion: Exposure apparently limited to residents of a 9 square block area. This exposure may have been a result of a gathering outside Bridgewater, exposure to a common source within Bridgewater, or be unassociated with a common gathering.
  2. Table: Place employed/occupation or school
     a) School associations (20 cases)
        (1) 20/30 or 66.7 percent of cases associated with schools
        (2) 19/30 or 63.3 percent of cases occurred among students
        (3) 1 case was a teacher

b) Others (10 cases); 10/30 or 33.3 percent of the cases were occupationally diverse

c) Limitations: Comparison of risk by place employed/occupation category not possible without population data

d) Conclusion: There appears to be an association between schools and the occurrence of cases. No cases occurred among students attending Bridgewater schools who lived outside of Bridgewater. However, the striking cluster of all categories by place of residence and the absence of cases in students living outside of Bridgewater would indicate that the association with schools may not be directly related to the circumstances leading to exposure.

C. Person

1. Table: Age and sex

a) The overall attack rate for Bridgewater was 2.1 cases per 1,000 population

b) Cases were distributed throughout all age groups with the exception of children under 5 years (0–4)

c) The attack rate among the affected age groupings (5–20+) was 2.3 cases per 1,000 population

d) The highest attack rate (4.0) occurred among the age group 10–14, with the next highest in the age group 5–9 (3.5)

e) The attack rate for the 5–14 year olds was 3.8 cases per 1,000 population

f) Limitations

(1) Neither total nor age-specific attack rates by sex can be calculated

(2) The apparent differentials in attack rates should be subjected to statistical tests of significance before firm conclusions can be drawn regarding true differentials in risk

(3) The risk of illness among the population 20 years of age and greater cannot be clearly established, since all 10 cases in this category occurred among individuals 22–43 years of age. The population 44 years of age and greater were apparently not at risk of illness

2. Calculation of ratio of attack rates. The attack rate (risk of acquiring illness) among persons 10 to 14 years old was 2.4 times greater than the attack rate (risk of acquiring disease) among persons in the remaining population of Bridgewater.

3. Calculation of mean and median ages

a) The median ages of both sexes are the same, 14.0 years

    b) The mean age of the female cases (18.9 years) is 1.2 times greater than the mean age of the male cases (15.8)

    c) Conclusion: The ages of the male and female cases are not significantly different

4. Conclusion: The distribution of cases by age and sex is compatible with common source exposure to hepatitis A virus. Of the various sources, food or water would seem most likely, although others cannot be ruled out at this point.

Hypothesis

A. The most likely disease is hepatitis A
   1. Incubation periods compatible (if exposure occurred on February 5 or 6)
   2. Duration of epidemic is compatible (exposure on February 5 or 6)
   3. Geographic cluster, school association, and age-sex distribution are also consistent
   4. Absence of cases in 0–4 age group may reflect lack of exposure to virus or inapparent infections that were not detected
B. Common source
   1. Duration of epidemic is 23 days
   2. Exposure of cases on February 5 or 6
   3. Some later cases could be a result of person-to-person spread. Exposure histories would be the only way to resolve this issue.
C. Vehicle: Food, water, or milk
D. Exposure on or about February 5 or 6
   1. Based primarily on information concerning the relatives of case #21 and the following assumptions
      a) The illnesses are etiologically similar to those of the resident cases
      b) Exposure of the relatives occurred during their visit to Bridgewater
   2. Exposure easily may have occurred in or around the affected blocks of residence in association with a common gathering or an individual exposure to a common source outside of such a gathering. The possibility of a gathering somewhere else in Bridgewater or even outside the city itself cannot be dismissed.

Hypothesis Testing

A. Establish a diagnosis—clinical and laboratory data
   1. Relatives of case #21

2. Bridgewater resident cases
3. Establish criteria to define an epidemic-associated case
B. Source
   1. If relatives of case #21 are considered epidemic-associated cases
     a) Establish activities during visit on February 5 or 6
     b) Identify exposure to potential sources of infection that also might be common to cases among residents
     c) If common gathering identified, then
       (1) Determine persons present
       (2) Determine potential sources of infection
       (3) Search for additional cases among others present
       (4) Obtain and compare exposure histories of cases and well persons in attendance
       (5) Identify common source
       (6) Search for source of contamination and establish circumstances present to account for such contamination
       (7) Identify others who also might have been exposed to the same source under different circumstances and seek additional cases
       (8) Ensure that the source of infection is no longer present
     d) If a common gathering is not identified, then
       (1) Establish and compare exposure histories of resident cases and relatives of case #21
       (2) Identify common source of infection
       (3) Search for additional cases among others potentially exposed
       (4) Search for source of contamination and establish circumstances present to account for it
       (5) Ensure that the source of infection is no longer present
   2. If relatives of case #21 are not considered epidemic-associated cases, then steps similar to those listed previously would be taken, although possibly with more difficulty. The inquiry concerning exposure histories may have to cover the period from January 24–February 6 unless a common gathering could be identified to limit the interval of inquiry.
C. Mode of transmission: The mode of transmission would be established through identification of the common source of infection. Contact with previous cases may have led to person-to-person spread.
D. Period of exposure: Compare exposure histories of cases and well persons over time and search for additional cases among others also potentially exposed would enable limits to be established for the period of exposure